SAY GOOD-BYE TO HEADACHES

By
Devi S. Nambudripad,
M.D., D.C., L.Ac., Ph.D.

Author of
Say Good-Bye To Illness and
Say Goodbye to ... Series

This book has already revolutionized
THE PRACTICE OF MEDICINE

The doctor of the future will give no medicine,
But will interest his patients
In the care of the human frame, in diet,
And in the cause and prevention of disease
Thomas A. Edison

Published by
DELTA PUBLISHING COMPANY
6714 Beach Blvd.
Buena Park, CA 90621
(888)-890-0670, (714) 523-8900 Fax: (714)-523-3068
Web site: www.naet.com

DEDICATION

This book is dedicated to
all my patients who suffer from headaches and
anyone wishing to
get well through NAET®

First Edition, 2007

Library of Congress Control No: 2006930519

ISBN-13: 978-0-9759277-6-2
ISBN-10: 0-9759277-6-0
EAN -13: 9780975 927762

Printed in U.S.A.

Table of Contents

Chapter 1

Chapter 2

Chapter 3

ACKNOWLEDGMENT

I am deeply grateful to my husband, Kris Nambudripad, for his encouragement and assistance in my schooling and later, in the formulation of this project. Without his cooperation in researching reference work, revision of manuscripts, word processing and proofreading, it is doubtful whether this book would have ever been completed.

My sincere thanks also go to the many clients who have entrusted their care to me, for without them I would have had no case studies, no feedback, and certainly no extensive source of personal research upon which to base this book.

I am also deeply grateful to Sue Tanner, Karen Watts, Margaret Brazil, Jennifer Bentley, Kathy Singer, Cindy Ho, Elizbeth Bonay, Loraine Pixley, Toby Weiss, Terri weiss, Mike Taleb, Steve McNair, Amy Clute, Sister Rosemary, Meher Davies, Nancy Dorsey, Ileen Garcia, Jana Shane, Pam Benson, to name a few among many of my devoted patients, for believing in me and staying with me until they got rid of their headaches through a series of NAET® treatments. I am grateful to these enthusiastic group of patients who helped me develop effective NAET® by supporting my theory and helping me to conduct the ongoing detective work on them.

I also have to express my thanks to my son, Roy, who assisted me in many ways in the writing of this book.

Say Good-bye to Headaches

I would like to express my thanks to Robert Prince, M.D., who graciously volunteered to write a foreword for this book. Dr. Prince has been practicing NAET® for over a decade now with good success.

Laurie Teitelbaum, MS, Chi Yu, Fong Tien and many of my associates who wish to remain anonymous for assisting me with this work, and Mr. Roy at Delta Publishing for his printing expertise. I am deeply grateful for my professional training and the knowledge and skills acquired in classes and seminars on chiropractic and kinesiology at the Southern California University, in Whittier, California; the California Acupuncture College in Los Angeles; SAMRA University of Oriental Medicine, Los Angeles; University of Health Sciences, School of Medicine, Antigua; and the clinical experience received at the clinics attached to these colleges.

My special thanks also go to Mala Moosad, N.D., R.N., L.Ac., Ph.D., Mohan Moosad, M.S., N.D., L. Ac, who supported and stood by me from the very beginning of my NAET® discovery and on-going research. Mohan and Mala also helped me immensely by taking over my work at the clinic so that I could complete the book. I also would like to acknowledge my thanks to my dear mother for nourishing me emotionally and nutritionally since childhood until now. My heartfelt thanks also go to Margaret Wu and Barbara Cesmat, NAET® practitioners, who have dedicated their time to help desperate allergy sufferers by assisting me in many ways to promote my mission of making NAET® available to every needy person in the universe. I would also like to acknowledge my everlasting thanks to my office manager, Janna Gossen, who worked with me from the first day of my practice over two decades ago and to all the other staff members and all other NAET® practitioners who support me and stand with me to help more allergic victims find health through NAET®.

I would like to remember the late Dr. Richard F. Farquhar at Farquhar Chiropractic Clinic in Bellflower, California. I was a student of chiropractic and acupuncture when I was doing preceptor-ship with him. When I told him about my NAET® discovery, he tried the treatment on himself and was amazed with the results. Then he encouraged me to practice NAET® on all his patients. Because of his generosity, I had the opportunity to treat hundreds of patients soon after I discovered NAET®.

I am so delighted to express my sincere thanks to the Los Angeles College of Chiropractic for teaching different branches of holistic medicine like kinesiology and Sacrooccipital techniques along with chiropractic in our school and also providing the students with a sound knowledge in nutrition. Because of that I was able to combine the art of kinesiology, chiropractic and nutrition along with acupuncture/acupressure and develop NAET®. California Acupuncture College also taught me a few lessons in kinesiology along with the art and science of acupuncture. I do not have enough words to express my heartfelt thanks and appreciation to California Acupuncture State Board for supporting NAET® from the beginning, permitting me to teach other licensed acupuncturists, by instantly making me a CEU provider soon after I discovered it. Perhaps the California Acupuncture State Board will never know how much they have helped humanity by validating my new technique and allowing me to share the treatment method with other practitioners and, through them, to the countless number of patients who now live a normal life. I am forever indebted to acupuncture and Oriental medicine. Without this knowledge, I, myself, would still be living in pain. Thank you for allowing me to share my experience with the world!

I also extend my sincere appreciation and thanks to my medical school professors for willing to part with their knowledge and help us become great physicians. I would like to extend my sincere thanks to these great teachers especially to my medical school mentors and professors from Antigua and from California, and the staff of the respective hospitals where I did my clinicals. Without their guidance and teaching I doubt if I could have completed the medical school.

All my mentors from all professional schools I attended have helped me to grow immensely at all levels. They are also indirectly responsible for the improvement of my personal health as well as that of my family, patients, and the health of other NAET® practitioners and their countless patients.

Many of my professors, doctors of Western and Oriental medicine, allopathy, chiropractic, kinesiology, as well as nutritional medicine, were willing to give of themselves by teaching and committing personal time, through interviews, to help me complete this book. I will always be eternally grateful to them. They demonstrated the highest ideals of the medical profession.

Devi S. Nambudripad,
M.D., D.C., L.Ac., Ph.D.(Acu.)

FOREWORD

By
Robert M. Prince, MD

Almost ten years ago, I received my first introduction to NAET. Several of our church members had had good results when they and their children had NAET® treatments by a local chiropractor in Charlotte, NC. They asked if some of our group might be able to obtain NAET® training to make this novel treatment available to family and church members. One of the ladies had a little girl who was still in diapers at the time and would have terribly messy diapers every time she ate anything with egg in it. The child had been desensitized to egg mix with NAET® treatments after which she had no more problems with eating eggs. I am a Medical Doctor, specializing in Psychiatry and my wife is a Registered Nurse. Both of us were steeped in traditional allopathic medical principles, which made us especially leery of anything as non-traditional as NAET®. However, we knew that it would be next to impossible to fool a child with any placebo treatment, so we were willing to look more closely at this alternative type of treatment.

Over the next few months, we went from being the greatest skeptics about NAET® to being some of it's greatest supporters. The reason is simply this – it works!

Three members of our group went for initial training by Dr. Devi Nambudripad ("Dr. Devi" as her students and patients fondly call her.) Three other persons from our group went to

California for this training several months later. I was very impressed with Dr. Devi and was quite fascinated with the report of her numerous successes in her book, <u>Say Goodbye to Illness</u>. But I still had a few lingering doubts after we returned from our initial training. Because of my doubts, I decided to put NAET® to the test by receiving a treatment for poison oak, a substance to which I had always been terribly allergic. My allergy was confirmed with the use of kinesiology (muscle testing of my arm.). I then was treated with acupressure tapping on selected acupuncture points along my spine while I held a jar of poison oak leaves in my hand (the standard non-invasive NAET® desensitization.) A few days later, I decided to put NAET® to the test. I took a Weed Eater to the back of our property and began vigorously clearing an area that was covered with poison oak. I knew from past experience that my usual result would be severe breaking out and itching within two or three days, so I took my chances and watched to see what would happen. After a couple of days, I felt a small lesion developing on the back of my neck, so my first thought was, "This thing is not working." But that one spot quickly dried up and that was it. Since that experience, I have had no adverse reaction to contact with poison oak leaves, and no further doubts that NAET® really does work!!

There have been some rare times when NAET® did not work as expected. Then we often have found that there can be an underlying emotional blockage sabotaging success. If these issues are examined and cleared, very often wonderful things happen..

One of my first observations while using NAET® to clear allergens was the amazing ability of NAET® to desensitize numerous individuals of allergies to foods, which they had been avoiding for years due to their adverse reactions. I was aware that standard allergy practices generally recognize no cure for food allergies other than avoiding the offending food. We soon began seeing many individuals who have been cleared of food allergies with very gratifying results. These include several children who, when cleared of their food allergens, found complete or almost complete relief from their regular stomachaches. A woman in her 60's was thrilled after NAET® treatments to be able to eat chocolate cake with her bridge club, after having had to leave off chocolate for years.

A man in his early forties came in with a long history of allergy to grains, also would get sick if he ingested chocolates, cheese or beer. He had been told by his doctors to stop eating a number of major food items, including dairy products, wheat, raw vegetables, and fruits. After he had been cleared of the first ten basic nutrients, using the NAET® protocol, he told us how pleased he was at being able to eat ice cream and fruit without adverse effects. After five more treatments, he was able to eat grains and tomatoes. He was especially thrilled to be able to consume pizza and beer while he and his family were on vacation.

A couple of years ago, we saw a middle-aged woman who had been treated with NAET® successfully four years earlier for allergies to eggs, milk, wheat, corn, nuts, and tomatoes. She had previously developed whelps when she consumed these items. On her return, she brought in a jar with cat fur and saliva, telling us that she had developed asthmatic symptoms after getting two house cats. When asked about her previous food allergies, she stated, "Oh, I can eat anything I want now." This last case, along with many others, helps to illustrate the long-lasting effect of NAET® treatments. They usually give permanent clearing of food allergies..

There was the very rewarding one time treatment of a very young nursing infant who was colicky and refusing to nurse. When treated for her mother's milk, the infant immediately was able to nurse comfortably, with mother and child being greatly pleased. Is it any wonder that I spoke at Dr. Devi's annual Symposium a few years ago on the topic, <u>NAET, THE ULTIMATE TREATMENT FOR FOOD ALLERGIES</u>

In our private clinic, NAET of Carolina, in Charlotte, we have been especially gratified with the results obtained with NAET® in treating autistic children. A five-year-old girl had developed normally until receiving some immunizations about age 2. After this she regressed severely and had never spoken in sentences, despite having a number of single words in her vocabulary. After she was diagnosed as being autistic, a doctor in Virginia told the parents that they could place her in an assisted living home when she was a little older, which was not at all what they wanted to hear. After she was treated for several of the basic allergens, they reported that on their way back home she went into the bathroom of their motel, turned on the light, brushed her teeth, used the bathroom, flushed the commode, and turned the light off. She did all these steps without any of the prompting she previously required. After she had completed approximately nine treatments, her parents were pleasantly surprised when she was playing with her little dog and said to it, "I eat you up." They were even more gratified when they told her, "We love you," and she responded, "I love you, too." These were the first sentences they had ever heard her say!

The parents of a young pre-school son were devastated to being told that he was autistic. They decided to bring him for regular NAET® treatments, even though their round-trip to Charlotte required over 5 hours of driving time. Since about age 2 he had been very limited in the number of foods which he could eat, had very limited verbal skills, made very little eye contact, and did quite a bit of "stimming." After receiving treatment for more than 25 allergens, they were very impressed with his progress. His mother wrote us that, "He is now eating a variety of foods. His verbal skills have improved. He makes better eye contact and he no longer 'stims.' This year our son is in a regular education kindergarten classroom . . . NAET® has changed our lives."

A research project in California compared 26 autistic children who received 50 NAET treatments during the year of 2005 with a group of randomly matched control cases, who had no NAET® treatments. Conclusions were drawn that NAET® treatments for the experimental subjects had significant improvements in their speech and communications when compared with the control subjects. Is it any wonder that I personally believe NAET® could well be the one of the most effective treatments available for autism?

Some of the most astounding results yet from the use of NAET® were reported at Dr. Devi's 12th Annual NAET® Symposium in July, 2006. Sister Naina is a Catholic nun who studied NAET® under Dr. Devi for a few months several years ago in California. She then returned to her job as principal of the Sophia Opportunity School in Bangalore, India, and has reported excellent results treating children in her school who had autism, ADHD, and other significant disorders having allergic manifestations. Her school is also associated with a charitable health clinic and orphanage. At the 2006 Symposium, she reported that persons who were unable or unwilling to care for the children any longer had dropped off a number of HIV positive infants and young children at the orphanage. Before using NAET®, the orphanage staff was reporting several deaths each month among this group of very unfortunate children. Sister Naina showed a video of a large group of these children who appeared critically ill, with multiple infections and weeping sores, prior to receiving NAET® treatments. The video showed these same children who were running around and playing happily after receiving a number of NAET® treatments. Lab data were presented on 6 of these children who were tested again for HIV after having received NAET® treatments for a year. She reported, "We didn't have enough money to test them more frequently." The astonishing results showed that all of these children had become HIV negative, with copies of the pre and post tests all documented and certified when these cases were presented to the professionals who were present at the Symposium. THESE CHILDREN AT ONE TIME WOULD NEVER HAVE BEEN CONSIDERED ELIGIBLE FOR ADOPTION BUT HAD NOW BECOME ELIGIBLE TO BE ADOPTED, WITH THE OPPORTUNITY TO LIVE A MUCH MORE PROMISING LIFE. THIS MARVELOUS GIFT WAS JUST ONE DRAMATIC EXAMPLE OF THE VALUE OF DR. DEVI'S DISCOVERY OF NAET.

In this volume, Dr. Devi follows the style of her previous outstanding book, Say Goodbye to Illness, giving multiple successful case studies of individuals who were greatly benefited by receiving NAET® for their headaches. She describes the different types of headaches and the procedures used by NAET® specialists in diagnosing and treating these symptoms which are often quite debilitating. She tells That headache is one of the leading causes of absence from work and that as many as 45 million Americans have chronic severe headaches that can at times be disabling.

The very first patient who came to our private NAET® clinic complained of having bad headaches every day when she taught school. That particular year, she was teaching in an older building - the previous year, in a new school building, she had no headaches. Since this was an acute case with her, my wife had instructed her to get a sample of the air from the schoolroom in which she was teaching. She was told to float a paper towel in a bowl of distilled water placed on top of a cabinet near her desk and to wait a couple of days for any toxic elements in the room to settle on that moist paper towel. She then put that wet paper towel in a jar and brought it to my office for testing. Kinesiology of her arm indicated she was definitely allergic to the substances in the jar. When she returned a week later, she said it was almost like a miracle - she had only one headache that week. That had occurred on a day when there had been a lot of chalk dust stirred up in the air near her desk. She brought in a piece of chalk for testing, and was quite allergic to it. After that treatment, we heard nothing more about her having headaches.

I would caution the reader that this case was much more straightforward than most headache cases. We had followed Dr. Devi's recommendation that we would be able to by-pass the usual basic protocol in treating this acute situation. Most people who have chronic headaches have more complex situations than this school teacher and get more lasting results from clearing the first 12-15 basic allergens as recommended by Dr. Devi.

Say Good-bye to Headaches

During the past 2 decades, Dr. Devi and her associates have trained over 9,000 health practitioners in the art of using NAET® to help alleviate the suffering of the numerous people who have chronic headaches, as well as other allergy-related disorders. These practitioners include many in this country in addition to many in Europe, Japan, India, Australia, and widely scattered areas all over the world. NAET® is not a "quick-fix", but statistics have shown that eighty percent of people with headaches diminish their symptoms and reduce the need for medication by the time they successfully complete treatment for 20 to 30 NAET basic groups of allergens

We encourage the readers of this newest book by Dr. Devi to experience this remarkable tool of NAET® to help them say GOODBYE TO HEADACHES.

Robert M. Prince, MD
NAET of North Carolina
Charlotte, NC

PREFACE

My mother suffered from frequent migraines for as long as I can remember. Later when I inquired, she told me that she began getting migraines at the age of thirteen or so. Initially as she recalled, her headaches used to be less frequent and less intense. As she got older she started getting them every three or four days. She took remedies from Western medicine as well as Ayurvedic herbal medicine regularly to control her migraines. No cause was found by either physicians (Western medical doctors or Ayurvedic physicians) for her malady. Some of her doctors thought that it was hormone-related and might get better after a childbirth. Instead of getting better she said her migraines got worse after childbirth in frequencies and intensities. According to her the only relief she received was from lying in a dark room with pin drop silence in the surroundings. Often she vomited after a couple of hours of head pain. That also gave her relief. Sometimes, very strong coffee gave her some relief.

She visited me in 1980 for a few months. The first two days of her visit she did not get any headaches. But on the third evening about 4:00 PM she began seeing flashes in front of her eyes. She said that the flashes such as these were the first warnings of her headaches. She was right. By 5:30 PM she was closed up in the bedroom with the curtains and shutters down. She even moved the alarm clock from the bedside table and put it in another room because the ticking sound of the clock bothered her. I sat next to her to apply cold compresses and give her a gentle head massage. I tiptoed in and out of the room. She had already taken the analgesics at the first sign of her headache. Even with that she did not get any relief. Her headache had to go through its stages. I watched her so helplessly and wished I could do something to ease her suffering. Finally by 9:00 PM she threw up. Then she slept.

The next morning she felt very tired. Other than that she was OK. She had no headache.

I did not want to see her suffer through another headache. I had to do something. I made an appointment with the best neurologist I knew in town. He examined her, did all necessary laboratory work, and scanned her head hoping to find a reason for her migraines. All the tests came back negative. The doctor said that my mother had classic migraines. He prescribed for her a stronger medication than the one she had been using. I was curious to know why she was getting headaches only every fourth day like clockwork? He had no answer to my puzzling question. The 4th day headaches remained a mystery.

She continued to have her every fourth-day migraines. She thought she was slightly better with the new prescription medication. In fact she said this medication was the only thing that helped her a bit so far. After three months she returned to India with a large supply of prescription medication that was somewhat helping her persistent migraines.

In 1983 I discovered NAET®. At that time, I was a senior student at the chiropractic college as well as at the acupuncture college. I attended chiropractic and acupuncture colleges simultaneously. I attended chiropractic in Whittier, California from 8:00 AM until 4:00 PM; then I attended the California Acupuncture Ccollege in Westwood near UCLA (35 miles away from the chiropractic college) from 5:00 PM until 10 PM. My classmate, and friend, Steven and I car-pooled together the 35-miles one way trip from Whittier to Westwood five days a week. After leaving chiropractic school, we found our way through the peak-hour Santa Monica traffic and arrived at the acupuncture college before the class started at 5:00 pm. Steven was a good driver and often we made it to the class on time.

Towards the final semester at the chiropractic school, I was selected to join Dr. R. Farquhar at his Bellflower chiropractic clinic as a preceptor. A holistic practitioner, Dr. Farquhar was reaching the age of retirement, had a lot of time on his hands and enjoyed sharing his knowledge with the new students. I considered myself very fortunate to have been selected to work and study with him for the following six months. I learned all practical application of chiropractic with him at his clinic.

When I began working with Dr. Farquhar I still continued to suffer from fibromyalgia, headaches, lower backaches, insomnia, and general fatigue along many other minor ailments. The smell of certain foods made me very nauseated and sick and often gave me symptoms similar to anaphylaxis. Seeing my misery, Dr. Farquhar volunteered to give me chiropractic treatments daily, often two or three times a day during a particular workday. These treatments helped me a great deal. I was able to work through the day without much discomfort.

Kathy K. was a regular patient for 30 years at the clinic. Around Halloween time in 1983, she brought some homemade wheat-pumpkin muffins to the clinic for the staff. Everybody said they were very delicious and asked me to try one. I was hesitant not knowing well my unpredictable reactions to foods. The doctor informed me that Kathy was very careful not to use any artificial coloring, food additives or food chemicals in her cooking. She always used organically grown natural ingredients and made everything from scratch. I told him that I was known to be severely allergic to wheat products in the past but he assured me that the reactions are usually not from the wheat but from the additives and I should be OK with Kathy's muffins. I took one small bite of the muffin first, it tasted really yummy. I waited for a few seconds and felt OK. So I took another bite. Before I swallowed it I felt like the room was spinning around me and in the next second I fell to the floor.

When I woke up I was lying on the table, the doctor was rubbing on the acupressure points around my naval and the staff was standing around the table. The doctor told me that I fainted after eating the muffin. He said I almost had an anaphylactic reaction to the wheat. They were ready to call 911 but I responded to the adrenal stimulation technique (a kinesiological technique) he used on me. They didn't have to call for emergency help.

After I recovered from that episode, I expressed my desire to learn everything about kinesiology, especially the adrenal stimulation technique. He agreed to teach me whatever he knows. Then he suggested for me to attend some classes with Dr. George Goodheart, the Guru of Kinesiology.

I was planning to take classes with Dr. Goodheat in the following January since he did not offer any classes until then. But as the fate would have the upper hand, I discovered NAET® on the 22nd of November, 1983. Following that discovery I became very busy treating all my allergies and my family's allergies. I was still attending full time acupuncture college at that time as well as doing 30 hours a week preceptorship at Farquhars. I didn't have any free time left to attend Dr. Goodheart's classes.

I treated most of my food allergies by the end of January of 1984. Because of the treatments I was able to eat most foods without much of a reaction.

Then one day I shared my NAET® discovery with Dr. Farquhar. I told him that at first I couldn't believe that my food reactions could go away. I was trying to convince myself that what I had discovered was for real. That's why I waited for eight weeks before I told him about it. I told him that I could eat most foods without getting sick including the wheat-pumpkin muffin. He stared at me in disbelief first. Then he laughed and said: You don't have to prove it to me by eating a wheat muffin. I believe you. Everything is possible in this world for those people who have determination and set your mind to what you want. You are one of those people and I have known it from the first time I saw you at the interview. That's why I chose you to be my student-preceptor. It takes an extraordinary person to attend two full time professional schools simultaneously, do well at schools, manage a household, take good care of a husband and a toddler. I am very proud of you. I shall be your first guinea pig.

I was flattered by his remarks. I knew he liked me from the very beginning but I had no idea he was able to look into the future. I thanked him for his confidence in me Then I asked him humbly, "Do you have any allergies? What can I treat you for? How can I demonstrate NAET® on you?"

Say Good-bye to Headaches

He showed me his left elbow-crease. He had a dollar size silvery, scaly, dry skin problem in that area. He said it was very itchy and he was tired of it. He had it there for over six years. He had tried everything and nothing had made any difference. He applied cortisone cream topically which gave him some relief for a short period. If you can cure this you don't need to do anything else to make me a believer.

I had no clue what his scaley patch of skin was from. "God, please help me, " silently I asked my God to guide me to help this man who had blind faith in me. I didn't want to disappoint him.

I examined the affected area, then I examined the corresponding acupuncture meridian. I located a couple of sensitive acupuncture points on his body related to the affected meridian. After doing a few more evaluations on those points I told him that skin problem was probably due to taking a vitamin supplement on a regular basis. I inquired if he had any complaints of a dull headache on the top of his head (vertex), constipation or low libido. His eyes widened with amazement. "You are right on the button," he said, "I have all those problems!"

He gave me a list of vitamins he was taking. I found him to be allergic to only one of them, "Orchex" the vitamin supplement from the Standard Process vitamin company. Doctor Farquhar had started taking this supplement six years ago after attending one of their product line seminars to increase his libido. I suggested that he stop taking it for a week and observe the body response from avoiding it. If we notice any reduction in itching, then we will know for sure this vitamin supplement is causing it. Then I would treat him with my new treatment and see the result. He agreed to go with my idea. Five days later he stopped having the episodes of headaches, stopped itching at the affected area, the scales peeled off and smooth skin began forming in the area. He was very pleased about the outcome from staying away from the vitamin and he said he didn't need to take it again. I reminded him that we were going to demonstrate NAET® on him. So the idea was to treat the allergy and use the supplement again to get the benefit. Avoiding was like running away from the problem and that was not the NAET® solution. He agreed to treat it with NAET®. He took three treatments on consecutive days to complete the treatments for "Orchex."

After completing the treatments satisfactorily, I suggested that he resume taking the supplement as before. We watched his response closely for a month. The supplement did not trigger any more headaches, skin problems or constipation but his libido did not increase. So I suggested that he add a certain Chinese prescription herbal formula along with "Orchex" and to let me know the result. A month later he reported to me that his wife was very pleased about his taking the new supplement I suggested.

Dr. Farquhar was impressed with the NAET® results. He was treated for a few more known allergens. Then he asked me to treat some of his chronically sick patients. Some of them had suffered from severe migraines for a number of years. He was able to ease their problems temporarily but never made these problems go away for a long term. No one else could help these patients on a long term basis either. Dr. Farquhar had seen them three times a week for many years. He gave me a list of five patients who were his regular chiropractic patients for over thirty years.

Dr. Farquhar was a true, genuine healer, a healer who really wanted his patients to get well by any and all means; even if it meant calling for assistance from his student. I was deeply touched by his humility.

At that time, I was not sure if NAET® could help migraines or headaches. I knew it could eliminate allergies. Therefore, if the headaches were triggered by allergies, it was likely would go away with NAET®. In any case, I decided to accept the challenge.

As we were discussing, Marjory pulled her car into the parking lot. She was a 45-year-old school teacher, who suffered from migraines from the age of 18 soon after she began working as a school teacher. She still worked at the same local school. She came in to the office two times a week to get treated for her migraines. She often visited emergency rooms for the same reasons too. On that particular day she came in with an exploding kind of migraine on the top of her head, spreading into her eyes. She was nauseous and had not eaten since Friday. She had already gone to the emergency room twice since Friday but had not received much help. She kept her eyes closed throughout my examination. From my NAET® testing, I found that the cause of her frequent migraines was from an allergy to mulberry leaves. I was reluctant to tell her my findings. I couldn't understand why anyone would use mulberry leaves for anything. Even more surprising is that they were used twice a week regularly enough to trigger headaches, and I was especially surprised that the person who used it was a school teacher. If she was a gardener I would have understood. I thought to myself that probably gardening was her hobby. Finally I asked her, "Marjory, do you use mulberry leaves for anything?"

She seemed startled by this question. She lifted her head, opened her eyes and looked at me for a few seconds and then answered, "I use them a lot. I use them in the flower arrangements I do in the office, then I also use them in the lab to feed the silkworms. Do you think that is causing my migraines?"

I let out a sigh of relief. It was then I knew that my diagnosis was right.

I answered confidently. "Yes, I think your frequent migraines are triggered by contacting mulberry leaves regularly. You seem to be allergic to the mulberry leaf. Can you get me a leaf so that I can treat your allergy to the leaves and hopefully you will get relief from your migraines."

"Yes," she said. "I have a bunch in the car. I shall bring it in right away." In spite of her aching head, she sounded very enthusiastic and rushed out of the door to the car. In a few seconds she returned with a bunch of mulberry leaves. According to NAET® testing, she was very allergic to them. She was treated for the leaves right away. I applied acupuncture needles on the gate points and let her rest for 30 minutes. After 30 minutes when I entered the treatment room to remove the acupuncture needles, she was sound asleep. I woke her up and removed the needles. She sat up and she had a beaming smile on her face.

"I have not felt this great in years. My head is very clear now. No more headaches. Thank you for this magical treatment." She paused a little then added, "I am very hungry now. Do you think it is OK for me to have some food? I haven't eaten since Friday."

"Of course," I said. "You can go out and eat anything you want. Please come back after you have eaten. I shall check you once more before you leave this area."

Say Good-bye to Headaches

She went out to get some food and returned in a few minutes with a large bowl of minestrone soup.

"Is it OK to eat this soup?" She inquired. "I don't want to do anything to trigger my headaches again."

I tested her with NST for the soup. She tested very strong. She returned to the car to eat the soup.

The doctor had stepped out of the office for a few minutes. After an hour Marjory and the doctor walked in together. They both were laughing about something.

Then Marjory came to me. "I am back. It feels so good not to have that nagging headache. I feel so free now. I pray the headache will never return."

"I am with you, Marjory," I said. "I hope you will never get another headache, but we have to make sure that we treat all your known allergies. Often, other allergens can give you similar reactions. Please take a couple of days rest. Then if you like we can start some NAET® treatments to eliminate all your other allergies to insure that your migraines will never return."

"Doctor Farquhar already told me all about it and how these treatment work, etc. Not only me, but my whole family needs your help. You are going to see all of us starting Wednesday for your special treatment. The doctor said it is OK for you to treat my whole family."

"The doctor is very enthusiastic about these treatments and also getting all of you well. I am so fortunate to have met him and it is a great privilege to work under his guidance. I can't wait to start treating all your allergies and find out how much help people can receive from these treatments."

"I can't wait either," she said with a ray of hope in her eyes.

The twice-a-week-migraines said good-bye to Marjory after the treatment for mulberry leaves. She had many other food and environmental allergies. We treated them one-by-one and she remained healthy ever since.

Then I got news from my mother that her headaches were back. The prescription pills were not being effective anymore.

I advised my mother to come to Los Angeles for another visit. I told her about NAET® and that probably NAET® could help her headaches without drugs.

As soon as she heard the news she didn't waste any time. In about three weeks, both my parents arrived in LA.

She had brought three large suitcases full of things from my hometown. One suitcase was filled with homegrown tea and coffee packages.

"Why did you bring so much coffee and tea?" I inquired. "We get all these here."

"Not this good quality," she said. "These coffee beans are grown in our backyard, handpicked and dried in the shade."

"Not only that, this coffee is the only thing giving her some relief when she gets her migraines," my father said. "Nothing else seems to be working lately. So she is afraid to leave home without this coffee. This has become like a security blanket to her."

Say Good-bye to Headaches

Childhood memories flashed through my mind. We had a large row of coffee plants growing in the huge backyard. Some coffee beans were red and some were orange-yellowish when they ripened. I helped in picking the coffee. The ripened beans we kept for our use. We sold the rest of the beans to the vendors. It was fun picking the coffee plums, the redder the better... then cleaning them, drying them in the shade... roasting them, grinding them once a month... the days we would roast and grind them, the smell of the coffee would be all over the house. My mother also would be having one of her migraines by then. So I ended up grinding them and storing them in airtight glass bottles to last for a month. In a day or so my mother felt better. I never drank coffee. My father had light coffee. But my mother liked double shot "latte", at least two times a day. Then whenever she had headaches she drank more double shot latte. She could not go without coffee. The reason for growing coffee in the house was to help with her headaches. She drank several cups of strong coffee daily. We grew almost everything on our farm. So my father decided to grow coffee too to keep the expenses down. He often remarked, "We are spending way too much on coffee and where can you get better coffee beans than the ones grown in your own back-yard?"

"Mom, at what age did you begin these headaches?" Now Marjory and mulberry leaves flashed through my mind, then the coffee, roasting and grinding, and my mother down with migraines. "It must be the coffee doing it to her," my mind kept saying. I couldn't wait to test her for coffee.

"I didn't have any headaches before my marriage," she said recalling from her memory. "I got married at thirteen. About six months after my marriage I got my first headache. Then they came on and off. But for the past several years they have come very regularly, I get them at least two to three times a week."

"When did you start drinking coffee?" Was my next question.

In our households, children were not allowed to drink coffee. They drank milk. Girls got married very young. After the marriage they were considered to be grown up. Then they were allowed to drink coffee, one of the things adults did.

"Probably I was around thirteen or so when I started drinking coffee," she said. I had to prepare coffee for your father everyday, twice a day. First I didn't like the taste of it. Then later on somehow I took a liking for it and now I cannot survive without coffee."

I did not even have to test her for her coffee allergy to arrive at a diagnosis for her incurable migraines. Most often, a detailed, thorough history can help you find the right diagnosis to most problems, especially allergy-based disorders. But I decided to test her for her own coffee with NST. She was very allergic to the coffee. When I told her that the allergy to coffee was causing her migraines she didn't want to believe me. She said she wasn't going to give up coffee drinking now.

I treated her for the coffee right away and hid all coffee in the basement cabinet so that she couldn't find it and wouldn't be tempted to drink it during the 25-hour waiting period after the NAET® treatment. Craving for the substance treated during the 25-hour waiting period is sometimes very difficult for some people, especially if one is addicted to it. My mother was addicted to coffee. She couldn't go half a day without it.

Say Good-bye to Headaches

She was very restless through the day. A couple of times she thought she was seeing flashing in front of her eyes... that was one of the warning signs of approaching migraines for her. But they did not materialize into headaches. We saw three home video movies along with her that night. Finally she slept.

On the following morning she woke up very late. She couldn't make or drink coffee anyway, so she decided to sleep in. When she woke up around 10:00 AM, she still did not have any headache. Strangely enough she did not have a craving for coffee either. She chewed packets of sugarless gum.

My mother has not consumed coffee regularly ever since that treatment, which has now been many years. Her 40-year-old migraines bid good-bye to her...forever. She didn't even miss coffee.

Now she drinks one cup of light tea in the morning. Maybe once a month or so she may drink a cup of coffee with milk. But this do not trigger migraines in her anymore.

These two detailed case studies are given here for a reason. My goal is to make the reader understand that allergens that trigger headaches and migraines are sitting next to you. You need to look for them and find them. Once you find them, either avoid them or get treated by NAET®. With NAET® you can still use these substances once in a while without triggering the same old problems.

According to NAET® theory, most illnesses arise from our interactions with the substances around us–our bodies perceiving them to be toxins. We use the products thinking they are good for us. Somewhere along our lives, our bodies began seeing them as toxins. When these substances turn out to be toxins for us, when we suffer headaches and other illnesses when we use them, we become confused and helpless. Most of us find salvation from these reactions in a doctor's office. A smart doctor will refer to your reactions by familiar medical names like migraines, cluster headaches, etc. instead of calling us crazy (even though that was most likely what he was thinking but not cruel enough to tell us to our face).

This doctor may even recommend a medication that has helped his other patients who have had similar reactions. If we are lucky, our symptoms would be reduced or eliminated and we would feel better and continue with our lives until the next attack.

NAET® is a simple technique that involves art and science from various medical disciplines. According to NAET® theory, allergies are the result of energy blockages in the body that are triggered by contact with various allergens. These triggers may especially be the products you use in your everyday life. Using the testing methods described in Chapter 5, you can locate the cause of your headache in the privacy of your own home.

The above two cases can be misleading. It is not always one allergen causing the problem. In many people various allergies can trigger the same problem. Because of this factor, we encourage you to test and treat everything that is reactive from your surroundings.

In most cases, a person who gets treated with NAET® would feel better and better after each treatment. It may take a couple of years for a person to become desensitized to every item on their long list of allergens, but in most cases, the patient begins to feel better right after the first treatment.

Say Good-bye to Headaches

NAET® treatments prepare the brain to respond normally to the treated allergen. This does not mean that after treating for a harmful chemical, our body does not recognize that the chemical is dangerous or harmful. When the body encounters the treated chemical in the future, the body releases it without causing panic or turmoil in the body.

Without knowing what is an allergen and what is not an allergen, we continue to expose ourselves to harmful allergens many times every day. Continuous exposures and re-exposures to various allergens throughout one's daily life can aggravate the condition of the body further. In such people, the presence of an allergen can trigger immediate allergic reactions, usually attacking the weakest organ first. Eventually, the other organs will be affected as well.

To be most effective, the NAET® Basic-15 need to be treated one-by-one without straying out of the treatment order.

Treating the Basic-15 in the correct order is especially important for people with chronic headaches. This prevents excess stress on their systems, so that their already stressed-out immune system can be more calm and confident in order to heal back to normalcy.

I would feel gratified, indeed, if the up-to-date material compiled herein were to contribute to my readers achieving, maintaining and enjoying good health; and if, through readers in the healing profession, an even larger number of people were to receive the possible benefits of NAET®.

I have focused on the issues of various types of allergy-based headaches in this book. A complete evaluation of the body and head should be done to rule out other disorders or involvements. If every report returns as negative, then the best bet is "an allergy" as a root cause. It is best at this point to find an NAET® Specialist near by to find the cause of the allergy and to fix it.

I have published many books on allergies and NAET®. Most of my books carry descriptions of meridians, testing procedures and some self-help tips. The book, "Say Good-bye to Illness" is the melting pot for health-related information on many areas of health in a very concise form. In the companion books, I focus on particular health issues as each title states, as in "Headaches" because several of my patients requested I write such a book related to their particular health issue. The reason for such requests they said was that they regained their health through NAET® but were unable to explain it adequately to their friends and colleagues with similar problems. They were aware that NAET® can help with wide range of health problems since most health problems are allergy-based. If there was a book on a particular health problem, then they could help their friends understand NAET® better. Another arguement some of my patients have is this: even though NAET® treats most health problems unless we specifically write up on them, people do not understand. Some people do not care to read about other's problems. They only worry about themselves. I can certainly understand that.

Due to growing interest from my patients, I have written many books related to different health disorders to explain how these problems can be easily helped with this drugfree, noninvasive, painless holistic treatment. NAET® Testing procedures and treatments overlap with all health disorders. So, I have to repeat certain chapters and materials in each book because it did not feel right to give partial information in the specific book and advise the reader to buy other books to get full information. So if someone would like to know about NAET® and Headaches, they only have to buy this book. All pertaining information will be given here. Then of course, if they like to read other books to educate themselves or help other family or friends with different health issues, they could buy them later.

If anyone wishes to learn more about acupuncture meridians and the possible pathological symptoms, or to find out about detailed information on diagnostic testing and evaluations to detect allergies, please read my book "Say Good-bye to Illness". All of my books and other NAET® products are available on our website:www.naet.com. Alternatively, to further enhance your understanding, you may wish to pursue some of the other relevant books and articles listed in the bibliography at the conclusion of this book.

Stay Allergy-Free and Enjoy Better HEALTH!

Devi S. Nambudripad,
M.D., D.C., L.Ac., Ph.D.

INTRODUCTION

I t is your right to eat whatever food you get or like to eat and digest the food, assimilate it and absorb the essential nutrients from whatever you eat without any trouble. It is also your right to live healthy in whatever environment you live with whomever you live and be happy. If you are able to accomplish this, you can say that you are in a healthy condition. If you are not able to do this you need to have yourself checked out by an NAET® specialist.

People without having any firsthand knowledge of NAET® might get confused by the above statement. On the other hand anyone with some experience with NAET, would agree with me because that is what you can accomplish through NAET®: be healthy and be happy.

People have been suffering from various types of headaches for a long time, probably from the beginning of the human existence. No one really knew the actual cause of headaches. Most healthcare practitioners identify disorders according to the signs and symptoms exhibited by the patients. We have symptom-oriented treatments for patients to keep them calm. Symptomatic treatments work very well most of the time. When the symptoms are gone, the doctor is happy, the patients are happy. There are some situations when the symptomatic treatments may not work. Then the doctor is puzzled, patients are confused and disappointed. In today's world this scenario happens very frequently.

Say Good-bye to Headaches

NAET® is a non-invasive, drug free, natural solution to eliminate allergies of all types and intensities using a blend of selective energy balancing, testing and treatment procedures from acupuncture/acupressure, allopathy, chiropractic, Kinesiology, and nutritional disciplines of medicine to bring better health in a person.

NAET® theory believes that some software problems (a virus perhaps?) in your brain-computer is the cause of allergies and allergy-based headaches.

NAET® is a way to reprogram your brain to its original state. NAET® is the computer virus treatment to help your brain to remove the faulty programs and replace it with the correct ones.

NAET® stresses the importance of life-style changes. Consuming non-allergic foods and drinks, living in a non-allergic environment, using non-allergic materials, associating with non allergic people, getting adequate exercise, maintaining sound mental health, all this means life-style changes. It means giving up eating junk food, eating more nutritious meals and eliminating emotional conflicts and unhappy situations.

NAET® is not a magic cure for anything. It is pure hard work based on stone-hard Oriental medical theory. If you are not willing to work hard, if you expect a magic bullet to cure all your problems instantly, NAET® is not for you. If you are willing to work hard, willing to make changes in your life-style you can get relief of your headaches. I have treated various types of headaches with good success. I strongly believe from my past experience that most of the headaches we see among patients are arising from some allergies, may be from foods, environmental agents, chemicals and pets or people. If the patient's presenting headaches are not due to allergies then NAET is not the way to treat their problems.

The main application of NAET® is to remove the adverse reactions between your body and other substances around you and thus to provide your body with good nutrition, and enhance the natural ability to absorb, assimilate the necessary elements from the food and eliminate the unwanted and toxic materials when they get into the body by any means. NAET® advises you to test everything around you for possible allergy before you use anything new or consume a new food. If you are allergic to every ingredient in the diet, no matter how pure and clean the diet is, you will never feel healthy. Now using NAET® home-based testing procedures, you can detect if the item is good for you or bad for you before you use them. If the item is not good for you, you do not have to use that particular item, but you can get a substitute.

When you get treated for the known allergens with NAET®, you will not react to these allergens anymore with the future contacts. When you get them into the body, if the items are beneficial for the body, your body will process them in order to derive the benefits from them; but if the items are not useful to the body, body will throw them out through natural elimination process without creating havoc in the immune system.

With this book you can now understand how allergies affect you and produce headaches of all kinds. You may need to go to an NAET® practitioner for several sessions or do it yourself if you have only mild or hidden allergies. When you read this book, you will learn how allergies and allergy-related illness can now be controlled.

NAET® was developed by Dr. Devi S. Nambudripad, who has been treating patients with this technique since 1983, and teaching other health professionals how to administer it since 1989. To date, more than 9,000 licensed medical practitioners have been trained in NAET® procedures and are practicing all over the world. For more information on NAET® or for an NAET® practitioner near you, log on to the NAET® website: www.naet.com.

How Do I Know I Have Allergies?

If you experience any unusual physical, physiological or emotional symptoms without any obvious reason, you can suspect an allergy.

Who Should Use this Book?

Anyone who is suffering from allergies or allergy-related health disease or condition should read this book. This natural, non invasive technique is ideal to treat infants, children, grown-ups, old and debilitated people who suffer from mild to severe allergic reactions without altering their current plan of treatment. NAET® encourages the use of all medications, supplements or other therapies while going through the NAET® program. When the patient gets better, the patient's regular physician can reduce or alter the dosage of drugs.

How is this Book Organized?

Chapter 1-Explains all about the history of headaches.

Chapter 2-Describes categories of allergens

Chapter 3- Explains Nambudripad's Testing Techniques and gives you information on various other allergy testing techniques.

Chapter 4- Describes normal and abnormal functions of acupuncture meridians.

Chapter 5-Explains NST(NeuroMuscular Sensitivity testing) to detect allergies.

Chapter 6-Discusses a few of the self-testing and home-self -treatment procedures.

Chapter 7-A collection of NAET® testimonials are given here.

Glossary-   This section will help you to understand the appropriate meaning of the medical terminology used in this book.

Introduction

Resources-Provided to assist you in finding natural products and consultants to support you while you work with your allergies.

Bibliography- Since NAET® is an energy balancing treatment, supporting bibliography on this subject is hard to find. This book cannot be completed without mentioning valuable information on Oriental Medicine and acupuncture, because NAET® was developed from Oriental Medicine. Since NAET® uses basic information from allopathy, kinesiology and chiropractic, books explaining these subject are also given in the bibliography.

Index- A detailed index is included to help you locate your area of interest quickly and easily.

HELPFUL SUGGESTIONS TO THE PROSPECTIVE NAET® PATIENT

I. INTRODUCTION

The prospective NAET® patient is required to read Say Good-bye to Illness or Say Good-bye to Your Allergies or listen to the CD (Say Good-bye to your allergies" is available on CD now to help with the patients who are unable to read due to their sensitivities to paper and ink.) before coming for the first treatment. NAET® is a method that helps to balance energies in the body. According to Oriental medical theory, when one's body energies are maintained in a balanced state, one does not suffer from most health disorders that arise from an energy imbalance. According to NAET® theory, allergies cause energy imbalances in the energy meridians, also known as energy pathways. An energy blockage is the primary cause for any allergic reaction towards any substance. When the energy blockage from an allergen is removed via NAET®, that particular allergen has not been shown to produce adverse reactions in the body on future contacts. NAET® is a mild, energy balancing, noninvasive, gentle procedure. It has not been shown to cause any long-term adverse effects on anyone within the last twenty years. While going through NAET® treatments, patients should try to keep their symptoms under control by taking necessary medications, therapies or other modalities. The patient is required to seek care of a primary care physician while getting NAET® treatment. If you suffer from a specific problem, you should also seek care of an appropriate medical specialist to manage health needs related to your condition. NAET® is only an energy balancing treatment. NAET® is not a primary care procedure.

II. Before the First Treatment

1. When you arrive at the office, these guidelines will be provided to you or your guardian or caretaker. You (they) MUST read and comply with these rules before beginning the testing procedures.

2. You should bring in a copy of ALL previous medical records, laboratory and radiological reports. You will be required to complete the following forms in the office: Personal data information sheet, history forms, symptom-survey form, and a consent form.

3. If you have a history of anaphylactic reactions toward any allergen, you must tell the NAET® practitioner before beginning the tests. Doing so, your NAET® practitioner can take adequate precaution to prevent you from becoming anaphylactic during treatments.

4. If you have a history of ANAPHYLAXIS, you should inform your practitioner on the very first visit before beginning the testing and treatments. People with history of anaphylaxis should ALWAYS be treated through a surrogate. They should wash their hands or rub both hands together immediately after each treatment. If you have severe allergies or anaphylactic history on any basic group of allergens, (Egg, milk, wheat, fish, etc.) those aller-

gens should be treated after completing rest of the Basic Fifteen groups. People with anaphylaxis are not required to hold the sample during the 20-minute waiting period.

5. NAET® Anaphylactic protocol SHOULD be followed strictly while getting treated. Your NAET® practitioner will instruct you appropriately.

III. Before Each Treatment

6. PLEASE do not wear any perfume, perfumed powder, strong smelling deodorant, hair spray, or after-shave and do not eat strong smelling herbs like raw garlic, seafood, etc., when coming to the NAET® clinic for treatments. If you suspect something is responsible for causing an allergic reaction, you may bring the item to the NAET® office in a thin glass container with a lid (as in a baby food jar with lid), wrapped in brown paper or a brown paper bag. Please do not bring items in plastic containers. Plastic containers cannot be used in testing.

7. There is NO smoking allowed in or around the office. PLEASE take a shower before you come for a treatment, and wear clean clothes to avoid smells of herbs, spices, perspiration, etc. Various smells can cause irritation and reactions in other sensitive patients in the clinic waiting room. Please do not eat or drink in the office. Another patient in the office waiting room might react to the smell of your food.

8. Wear minimum or no jewelry when you come in for a treatment. Avoid wearing large crystals or large diamonds. NAET can be done while wearing your own clothes provided you wear simple, loose clothes without ANY art work or embroidery with crystals, beads, stones, metals, glass or plastic pieces. It is fine to wear simple wrist watches while testing or treatments. Avoid watches with sharp needles, cell phones, calculators, tape recorders, photo camera, etc.

9. PLEASE do not wear any guns or knives to the office even when they are part of your job requirements. Please do NOT bring sharp metal objects, large keys, sharp toys, heavy toys, or toy guns to the office.

10. Please turn off your cell phones inside the waiting room and in the treatment room. Other sensitive patients might react to your cell phone. Cell phones should be off and kept away from your body during NAET® testing and desensitization treatment.

11. ALWAYS eat before you come for the treatment. You should not take NAET® treatments and acupuncture when you are hungry. If you have a long wait in your practitioner's office, please bring a snack with you, leave it in the car or outside the office. Five to ten minutes before your treatment, please go outside the clinic and eat your food, wash your hands with soap and water, and rinse your mouth before you return to the clinic for the treatment.

12. Please WASH your hands with soap and water before beginning the Neuromuscular sensitivity testing procedure (NST). Hand-washing will remove any residue left on your hands from other substances.

13. Do NOT treat with NAET® if you are extremely tired, worked a night shift, or worked too many hours without a break.

IV. During Each Treatment

14. You should NOT have any companion with you standing or sitting within your magnetic field during treatment. You should not bring any children or pets to the treatment room while you are being treated. You should be alone with your NAET® practitioner while you get tested or treated with NAET®.

15. Since NAET® is a mind-body balancing procedure, the NAET® practitioner needs to receive permission from your con-

scious and subconscious minds before performing any energy balancing procedures. Signing the consent is the permission from the conscious mind. But permission from the subconscious is necessary for a successful NAET treatment. For a trained practitioner it takes only a few seconds to seek permission from the subconscious. In rare occasions, it has been shown that certain person's subconscious mind does not grant permission to perform NAET® testing or treatment. In such cases, the NAET® practitioner may NOT proceed with NAET® testing. Instead the NAET® practitioner will make appropriate referrals for further evaluations related to their health conditions.

16. The NAET® practitioner must get permission from YOUR subconscious mind before each NAET® desensitization treatment as well. On a particular visit, if your brain did not give favorable signals for a new treatment, you will be rescheduled for another date. This is for your best benefit. It has been shown that even anaphylactic cases also can be treated successfully for the anaphylaxis-producing allergen when the NAET® practitioner gets permission from the patient's brain before doing the treatment. You may rest for a few days until your brain and body are ready to get more treatments or you may be able to receive other immune system supporting treatments like chiropractic adjustments, acupuncture, massage, Yoga, etc. while waiting.

17. While performing NST, the patient SHOULD wash or rub his/her hands together for 30 seconds between touching different samples. The energy of the previously tested sample has shown to produce false results if the energy of the previous item has not been removed from the hands before touching a new one.

18. While receiving NST testing or NAET® desensitization procedures PLEASE make a loose fist with your free hand (one without the allergen) in order to prevent contact between the table or your clothes with your fingers while testing.

19. Do not eat or chew gum or candy DURING NST testing or NAET® treatment.

20. The NAET® practitioner will not have ANYONE observing the treatment or taking notes, from a close proximity. The distance varies with each patient for each allergen. Your practitioner will know how to determine the distance.

21. If you are unable to test yourself (if you are a child, old person, too strong, too weak, disabled, advanced stage of pregnancy, etc.), then you SHOULD be tested through a surrogate so that the practitioner can get accurate information about your sensitivities. You should maintain skin-to-skin contact with the surrogate during testing and the surrogate should rub his/her hands together or wash hands between testing different allergens.

22. You could also be treated through a surrogate's body and get the exact benefit as if you were getting treated directly. Patients in advanced stage of pregnancy, morbidly obese, with psoriasis or other debilitating skin problem, back surgery, scoliosis, or a history of anaphylaxis, etc., SHOULD receive NAET® treatments through a surrogate.

V. The Basic 15 treatments

23. The NAET Basic 15 treatments are in fact the basic essential nutrients for everyone. If you are allergic to them your body may not receive adequate nutrients. That will cause to lower the immune system function and may cause to have various health disorders due to nutritional deficiencies brought on by allergies. When your immune system is maintained at a normal level, not only you feel better overall, your allergic sensitivity will be reduced with the result, you need fewer NAET treatments to get maximum results.

VI. Reasons Why Treatments May Need to be Given Out of Order

24. If you have allergies to white rice, or pasta, they can be treated before the Basic treatments.

25. Hard-to-avoid items like prescription drugs should be treated first in the doctor's office, then treated at home through self-treatment every two hours. In case of a drug that cannot be avoided, you should treat by gate-massage before and after you take the drug as well as massaging the gates every two hours for the 25 hours after the initial treatment.

26. When a patient has an ACUTE problem, practitioners will treat the acute problem before resuming the normal order of treatments if the patient's brain gives permission to do so. For instance, when a patient is reacting to a particular food that was eaten recently, a medication that is essential for the patient's survival (like pain medication, cortisone, antihistamine, antidepressants, heart medication, etc.), fire-smoke, accidental exposure to fumes, drinking water, city water, acute emotional imbalances like the death of a loved one, etc., can be treated as an acute allergen before completing the basic fifteen treatments as long as the body permits. If someone has severe reaction to pollens, weeds, cigarette smoke, regular drugs like chemotherapy drugs, antibiotics, standard emotional blockage removal treatments, person-to-person allergies, etc., can be treated after completing six basic treatments (after completing sugar mix). When the treatment for acute allergen is completed satisfactorily, you should go back to the basics and continue as before.

VII. After Treatments

27. You must wash your hands with plain water after treatment BEFORE you leave the office. After the treatment if you

cannot wash or rinse your hands, vigorously rubbing your hands by interlacing your fingers for 30 seconds will be sufficient.

28. After the NAET® desensitization, PLEASE do not exercise vigorously for 6 hours. A mild walk is fine.

29. AVOID exposure to extreme hot or cold temperature after the desensitization treatment.

30. Do NOT bathe or shower for 6 hours following the NAET® treatment.

31. Do not read or touch other objects with your FINGERS during the 20 minutes waiting period after NAET® treatment.

32. Do NOT cross your hands or feet during the first 20 minutes following the NAET® treatment. Lying or resting with a calm mind will be beneficial. You could visualize positive, warm energy circulation through the 12 meridians while resting. Meditation is allowed. After an emotional NAET®, you are advised to think positively during the 20 minute waiting period about the issue which was treated.

33. Your practitioner WILL ask you to avoid the treated allergen for 25 hours or more as indicated by his/her testing after the completion of the treatment in the office. After the treatment you should avoid eating, touching, breathing and coming within 5 feet of the substance that was treated following 25 hours after treatment. It is also suggested after completing your treatment satisfactorily for an allergen, that you consume a small amount of the item daily for three to four days. If the treatment is not completely finished, you will bring out some minor symptoms and your practitioner can investigate the reasons behind those symptoms and eliminate them. Another benefit of introducing the treated allergen into your body is to reconfirm the brain and nervous system about the harmlessness of the item so that your nervous system will not forget about this allergen in the future even if you never ate them later for years.

34. It is highly recommended that after three NAET® basic treatments, you TRY to consume foods and drinks from the desensitized groups only. Add new items to your list as you complete each treatment. This will reduce your overall discomfort while going through the rest of the treatments and your NAET® treatments will be more effective and you will be able to see results with NAET® faster. Depending on your immune system the treatments can be scheduled. A patient with severe allergies and poor immune system can only tolerate one treatment per week. But patients with better immune system have shown to tolerate three or more treatments per week. Your practitioner can test your body for the appropriate treatment plan.

35. If you are a highly SENSITIVE person, or if you experience any discomfort during the 25 hour-avoidance period after the treatment (crying spells, depression, unusual emotions or unusual pains anywhere in the body, etc.), you may need to balance your gates every two hours on your own at home while you are AWAKE. When you sleep, you do not need to set an alarm to wake you every two hours. Instead whenever you wake up, you can continue treating again.

36. The practitioner can determine the APPROXIMATE number of hours of avoidance by using question response testing for patients who have difficulty avoiding food for 25 hours. Infants and children can be treated in the evening or before going to sleep for hard-to-avoid items. Please ask your practitioner if you have questions.

37. If someone has a hard time avoiding the allergen for a specific amount of time for any particular reason, he/she should BALANCE his/her gate points every two hours as well as before and after exposure to the allergen. In case the patient has developmental disabilities, caretakers should be instructed to massage the gate points (Read Page 58 in the book, Living Pain Free by the author) every two hours during the 25 hours and also before and

after touching the treated allergen. Your practitioner will teach you the self-balancing technique if you do not understand by reading the book, Living Pain Free. It is advisable for you to BUY this self-help book with Illustrations since it can help you to control or reduce various allergic reactions and discomforts arising from untreated allergies by massaging the appropriate acupressure self-treatment points whenever the need arises.

38. No adverse reactions have been noted when a person eats food INCLUDING the food he/she was treated, for 20 minutes following the retest of the initial treatment for the allergen. The 25 hour-restriction begins 30 minutes after the completion of the treatment. Do not eat HEAVY meals before or after the NAET® or acupuncture treatments, but DRINK a glass of water before the NAET® treatment. Energy moves better in a well hydrated body. Drink 4-6 glasses of water through the day after NAET® treatments to help flush out the toxins produced during the treatment.

39. You are advised to MAINTAIN your own treatment and food diary in The Guide Book after each treatment. Write down all the good and bad symptoms you experience during 25 hours following treatment and bring it to your practitioner on your next visit. If you have frequent health problems and you do not know the cause of your problems, write down your daily activities for a month in a separate notebook. Record all the food and drinks you consumed even if they were in small portions and record also anything new you have purchased in the house or work area since the problem started. Bring your record to the office and let your NAET® practitioner test you for the items in your list to find the culprit.

40. You may need to take EXTRA precaution while you get treated for environmental substances: (mineral mix, metals, water, leather, formaldehyde, fabric, wood, mold, mercury, newspaper, chemicals, flowers, etc.). Apart from staying away from these items, you may also need to wear a mask, gloves, socks, shoes,

gowns, scarves, earplugs, etc. You can also massage the gate points every two hours while awake during the 25-hour period if it is not completely avoidable.

41. During the 25 hours or afterwards, if you get a life-threatening reaction from an allergen (either from the one you were treated in the office or another one), you MUST seek emergency help immediately from a primary care physician or emergency room, or by calling 911.

42. Once every month or so, or after completing treatments for TEN to FIFTEEN allergens, your practitioner will repeat NST on all treated allergens. If an allergen wasn't passing over 50 percent at the time, they will be boosted up again. No avoidance is necessary at this time.

43. AFTER the Basic Fifteen treatments with the practitioner, patient should begin to gather a small sample of every day food and drinks and holding the sample, balance the gate points every night before bedtime.

44. DRINK one 6 ounce-glass of water first thing in the morning. Drink 1 glass of water before bedtime.

45. Remember to CHECK with your practitioner for the item you treated, after 25 hours, and at least within one week to make sure you have completed the treatment.

VIII. Additional Information about NAET®

46. NAET® is a HOLISTIC procedure. It balances the entire body including: physical, physiological and emotional functions. Everyone needs balance in all these levels of the body to be healthy. If one area is not balanced properly, other areas cannot function normally. NAET® emotional balancing procedure has been shown to produce marvelous results in people who suffer from environmental illness, chemical reactions, chronic pain disorders, other

chronic illnesses, autism and ADHD, etc. This emotional balancing treatment will be provided to the patient without additional cost if done in conjunction with a treatment for another substance. After completion of Sugar treatment (after completing six basic treatments), NAET® emotional balancing treatments can be administered upon request.

47. NAET® emotional balancing procedures do NOT replace the need for traditional psychological or psychiatric help. If you are getting treatments in these areas prior to NAET®, please continue with your therapies and medications as needed. If you for any reason do not like to be balanced emotionally by your NAET® practitioner (due to religious reasons, etc.), you should inform the NAET® practitioner on the initial visit, then emotional balancing procedure will be excluded from your treatment plan.

48 If you did not complete the treatment, or if you could not complete the specific NAET® treatment for some reason, do not panic. NAET® is a mild, energy balancing, noninvasive, gentle procedure. It has not been shown to cause any long-term adverse effects on anyone since its discovery within the last twenty-three years. Your temporary symptoms may be due to the incomplete treatment and may continue for up to two or three weeks maximum. Drink about 4-6 glasses of boiled cooled water daily to help with your energy circulation.

49. Eventually the particular symptoms will wear off and you may return to your pre-NAET® status if you did not repeat the treatment for the unfinished allergen. For example, if you suffered from insomnia prior to NAET® treatment, you may continue to have insomnia; if you suffered from pain disorders, you may continue to suffer from pain disorders, etc. An allergen which was treated halfway has not shown to render any benefit to the patient at all. Human body forgets and adapts to new ways fast. The incomplete treatment is forgotten in about three days to a week in most cases, but in some cases it has shown to take as long as three

weeks, then the body learns to focus on current events. Thus, in a few days, an incompletely treated allergen is usually viewed by the body as an allergen that has never been treated before.

50. But if you had to stop the NAET treatment for the particular allergen because you had no means to get to the office, then you can balance the energy for the particular item at home on your own by holding the item while massaging the gate points once every four hours while awake for two to three weeks or as short or as long as the body needs to view that as a friendly item. This method will only work after one has been treated initially with a trained practitioner, and the treatment was not completed for some reason. If it is an uncomplicated, individual item, like a piece of sourdough bread, a piece of meat, a hot dog, a laxative or a pain pill like Tylenol or another drug, a particular piece of fabric (a shirt, scarf), etc., then the patient or the caretaker can complete the treatment in this manner at home. CAUTION: this should be done only on a single allergen, never try on a group of allergens.

51. After completing treatment for an allergen, if NST tested strong on retest but the patient is still suffering from prior symptoms, the patient should be allowed to rest a few days to a couple of weeks without any new NAET® treatment. This is in fact to rule out or to determine if the desensitization towards the particular allergen was successful or not; and to determine if the presenting symptom is arising from another source or not. If the particular allergen treatment is incomplete, if you wait a few days the NST will produce a weak response either on its own or with some combinations. Then the treatment on the allergen itself or with a combination can be repeated at that time. While waiting to detect the outcome of the previous treatment, it is OK to boost up the immune system with acupuncture, chiropractic treatments, massages, herbs or other therapies. Or the patient can continue to self balance for the item at home as described above.

52. Sometimes, the patient continues to have the same symptom but NST does not show any weakness on the previously treated allergen. In such cases it has shown that the patient passed the treated allergen but another allergen capable of producing similar symptoms has been identified as the culprit. Usually people with history of allergies react to more than one or a few allergens. When one allergen gets desensitized and eliminated from the body, others will get noticed easier, hence the symptom of the previous allergen continues until all the allergens are desensitized with NAET®.

53. When one has a weakness in any particular area of the body, every allergen affects that area of the body giving rise to symptom similar to the first one. This pattern is especially noticed in patients with asthma, sinus problems, autistic disorders, attention-deficit hyperactive disorders, chronic pain syndrome, as in degenerative arthritis, fibromyalgia, lupus, headaches, migraines, backaches, myofascial pain, peripheral neuropathy, PMS, insomnia, manic or depressive disorders, etc. Because of this mechanism, until you complete NAET for Basic Fifteen, you may not see much changes in your health in these cases.

54. When you are allergic to a substance, your body produces lots of endogenous toxins. After you are treated to an allergen, it takes 24 hours for the body to detoxify the allergen from all 12 major meridians (each meridian takes 2 hours) naturally to get the toxins out of the body. SOME patients may not have 24 hour avoidance or restrictions. Some may pass the allergen right after the treatment; some may take just a few hours; some may take 25 hours, yet some others may take 40 hours. Even though NST demonstrated that you would clear the allergen in 10 minutes or so, it is to your advantage to avoid the item for the whole 25 hours (24 hours plus one hour guard-band) allowing the body to detox naturally. After a few NAET® treatments, you have the option to go on a good detoxification program using different products (herbs, minerals, etc.) to clean up your system. But if you faithfully follow

the 25-hour avoidance, you may not need any special detoxification since the body is able to naturally eliminate the toxins in time if given a chance.

55. You are advised to continue ALL medications and other treatment modalities as they have been prescribed unless otherwise directed by the doctors who prescribed them. PLEASE do not stop any other treatment you are on: medication, therapy, chiropractic treatments, massages, etc.

56. NAET® treatments have NOT been shown to interfere with any other treatment. In fact, if you can keep your body free of toxin accumulation and keep your symptoms under control by using medication or therapies, NAET® has shown to work better.

57. For FEMALE patients: Treatments are not advisable during the first three days of menstrual cycle.

58. NAET® treatments during pregnancy have not shown to cause any adverse effects to the mother or child so far. In fact tremendous benefits have been noted in both cases. When the mothers receive adequate NAET® treatments during pregnancy (at least 15 basics and all known allergens of the mother treated), their children are born with very few allergies when compared with their siblings who never had exposure to NAET® before birth.

59. When you go through the NAET® treatment program, you will be advised to get supplemented with appropriate amount of vitamins, minerals, and other nutrients for a while if it is indicated. When the nutrients are supplemented appropriately pain and discomfort arising from various disorders like chronic fatigue, general body aches, arthritis, and other pain disorders due to deficiencies, etc., will be reduced.

60. If you do not show any improvement in your health status after successfully passing Basic ten to fifteen allergen groups at all three levels, probably NAET® is not for you. Please ask your practitioner to refer you to another source of healthcare facility.

Say Good-bye to Headaches

CHAPTER 1

HISTORY OF HEADACHES

Humans have suffered from headache for centuries. Searching through the history of headaches, various interesting anecdotes and developments have been noted. Head pains are described in the Bible as well as in medical writings from ancient Egypt, Babylonia, Greece, Rome, India, and China. A common cure for headaches in ancient Egypt and India was to inhale the smoke from burning sandalwood.

Historical evidence from the 7th Century BC shows that severe chronic headaches were treated by the oldest known surgical procedure, known as trepanning or trephining, in which the surgeon drilled a hole as large as 1–2 inches in diameter in the patient's skull without benefit of anesthesia presumably to relieve the pressure and "evil spirits or demons" inside the head that might be causing such pain. Evidence of trepanning has been found in skulls from CroMagnon people that are about 40,000 years old. During the next several thousand years, descriptions of headache and various treatments for it continued in different ways in different cultures, which only shows even those days headaches were a universal ailment. People everywhere desperately were looking for cures for headaches either for themselves or to help their loved ones or to help their patients. The heart warming stories of such explorations can be found scattered throughout art, literature and primitive medical texts.

The recorded history of humanity's suffering from headache dates back to 9000 years ago when basic drastic therapy of that time was trepanation. Headache with neuralgia was recorded in the medical documents of the ancient Egyptians as early as 1200 BC. In 400 BC Hippocrates described the visual aura that can precede the migraine headache, and the relief that can be induced by vomiting.

Aretaeus of Cappodocia (2nd century AD) is often credited as the "discoverer" of migraine because of his classic descriptions of the condition. Some causes or triggers of migraine were recognized during this era. For example, Celsus (215-300 AD) correctly described what are now recognized as typical migraine triggers: "drinking wine, dyspepsia, cold, heat of fire, or the sun."

Galenus of Pergamon used the term "hemicrania", from which the word "migraine" was derived. He thought there was a connection between the stomach and the brain because of the nausea and vomiting that often accompany an attack. For relief of migraine, Spanish-born physician Abulcasis, also known as Abu El Quasim, suggested application of a hot iron to the head or insertion of garlic into an incision made in the temple. In the Medieval Ages migraine was recognized as a discrete medical disorder with treatment ranging from hot irons to blood letting and even witchcraft. Followers of Galenus explained migraine as caused by aggressive yellow bile. Avicenna described migraine in his textbook "El Qanoon fel teb" as "… small movements, drinking and eating, and sounds provoke the pain… the patient cannot tolerate the sound of speaking and light. He would like to rest in darkness alone". Abu Bakr Mohamed Ibn Zakariya Râzi noted the association of headache with different events in the lives of women, "...And such a headache may be observed after delivery and abortion or during menopause and dysmenorrhea".

Jean Nicot, a French diplomat, introduced tobacco to the French court. In 1560, while serving as ambassador in Portugal, he was shown a tobacco plant in the garden of Lisbon botanist Damião de Goes, who claimed it had healing properties. Nicot brought home seeds and leaves of tobacco, to try out its marvelous therapeutic value. He applied it to his nose and forehead and found it relieved his headaches. Nicot sent snuff to Catherine de Medici, the Queen of France to treat her migraine headaches. She was impressed with its results.

During much of human history, artistic, literary and medical descriptions of migraine or headache have focused on male sufferers, even though in ancient times as today, women with migraines undoubtedly outnumbered males with the disorder. A few descriptions of the disorder in women do survive, though. One of the most interesting is found in the writings of the 12th century Abbess and mystic Hildegarde of Bingen, presumably describing a migraine aura:

"I saw a great star, most splendid and beautiful, and with it an exceeding multitude of falling sparks with which the star followed southward...and suddenly they were all annihilated, being turned into black coals...and cast into the abyss so that I could see them no more."

In Bibliotheca Anatomica, Medic, Chirurgica, published in London in 1712, five major types of headaches are described, including the "Megrim," recognizable as classic migraine. Graham and Wolff (1938) published their paper advocating ergotamine tart for relieving migraine. Later in the 20th century, Harold Wolff (1950) developed the experimental approach to the study of headache and elaborated the vascular theory of migraine. The actual cause of head pains are still being debated among medical researchers.

STATISTICS ON HEADACHES

Headache is one of the leading causes of absence from work. Ranging from slight discomfort to total disability, headaches are a serious threat to health everywhere.

The American Council for Headache Education (ACHE) reports that, during the past year, nearly 90 percent of men and 95 percent of women have had at least one headache.

Eighteen percent of women and six percent of men suffer from migraines, a ratio of 3:1.

According to the National Institute of Neurological Disorders and Stroke (NINDS) and the American Council for Headache Education (ACHE): As many as 45 million Americans have chronic, severe headaches that can be disabling.

Headaches result in more than 8 million doctor visits a year.

Most people with a headache use nonprescription pain relievers to treat their symptoms. Because store shelves hold a vast array of pain relievers, and there is a growing trend towards self-care, Americans have a responsibility to examine facts about headaches and pain relievers.

According to estimates, approximately 29.5 million people in the United States suffer from migraines. Four out of five of them report a family history of migraine, but scientists are not sure if this is genetic or a family predisposition.

60% of people who have migraines have one or more severe attacks each month.

It is estimated that about 45-50 million a year seek medical help for headaches in America. Among them about 35 million people suffer from migraines. About 70% take painkillers at least once a month. 12.5 million Americans get a headache every day.

Migraine sufferers lose more than 157 million workdays because of headache pain.

UNDERSTANDING HEADACHES

WHAT IS A HEADACHE?

Headache is a pain felt anywhere in the head above the neck that may be a disorder on its own, a symptom of an underlying medical condition or functioning as a warning signal for more serious disorder(s). The medical term for headache is cephalalgia. Headache is one of the most common and universal human ailments, probably began since human life began in the world.

TYPES OF HEADACHES

PRIMARY HEADACHES

These types of headaches account for more than 90 percent of headaches, and include the following:

- ◆ **Migraine (Vascular) headaches**

  - Classic Migraine (with aura)

  - Common Migraine (without aura)

- ◆ **Other Types**

  - Hemiplegic migraine

  - Occular migraine

  - Basilar artery migraine

  - Headache-free migraine

  - Food sensitivities and food allergies

- Chemical and environmental sensitivities
- Hormone related
- Psychogenic causes
- Allergy to people

◆ Tension headaches

- **Episodic Tension Headaches**
- Stress
- Muscular contractions
- Torticollis
- Acute food allergies or food poisoning

- **Chronic Tension Headaches**
- Musculo-skeletal problems of upper back
- Affer-effect of whiplash
- Chemical and environmental sensitivities

◆ **Cluster headaches**

- Episodic Cluster Headaches
- Chronic Cluster Headaches
- Toxic Headaches
- Hypertensive Headaches
- Rebound Headaches

SECONDARY HEADACHES

◆ Traction headaches

- Brain tumors

- Aneurysm

- Hydrocephalus

◆ Inflammatory headaches

- Meningitis

- Head Injury

- Temporal arteritis

- Stroke

- Lumbar puncture

- Sinus infections

- Referred Headache

- Idiopathic intracranial hypertension

- Exertion

- Dental

- Temporomandibular joint disorder

CAUSES OF HEADACHES IN GENERAL

- Nerve Irritation

The major cause of headache is due to nerve irritation. Nerves get irritated in the parts above the neck leading to pain.

- Headaches Due To Upper Respiratory Infections

Examples are: fever, cold, flu, cough, etc. During infections, the body encourages more blood and lymph to flow to the affected area in the pretext to float away the causative agent of the infection. This excess blood circulation causes the tissue to swell up thus producing nerve irritation and resulting pain in the swollen tissue and in the surrounded area.

- Headaches due to hormonal imbalances

Premenstrual syndrome, pregnancy, menopause, andropause, etc. can act as triggers for headaches. In these cases, the person may be allergic to their own hormones.

- Headaches due to stress, insomnia, and stress-related issues.

- Headaches due to psychogenic causes

- Headaches due to inappropriate nutritional intake (Hypoglycemia, etc.)

- Headaches due to metabolic disorders (Thyroid, diabetes, kidney disorders, etc.)

- Headaches due to hypertensive disorders, cardiovascular and circulatory disorders, etc. (Stroke, TIAs, etc.)

- Headaches from toxic overload in the body (Constipation, improper elimination, etc.)

- Headaches due to nutritional deficiencies (lack of essential vitamins, minerals, proteins, etc.)

- Headaches due to sensitivities and allergies to daily essential nutrition (food allergies)
- Headaches due to allergies and sensitivities to chemicals and environmental agents (fabrics, fabric detergent, pillow, pillow cases, dry cleaning agents, carbon monoxide poisoning, exposure to extreme heat, cold, etc.)
- Headaches due to allergy to pets
- Headaches due to allergies to people
- Headaches due to acute or chronic traumas and injuries (cerebral concussion, old or new auto accidents, whiplash injuries, sports injuries, etc.)
- Headaches due to organic causes (brain tumors, aneurysm, etc.)
- Headaches due to brain infections like meningitis, encephalitis, etc.
- Headaches due to intoxication (alcohol, overeating, etc.)
- Headaches due to toxins from Substance abuse

DIAGNOSIS OF HEADACHES IN GENERAL

- A detailed medical history (should include past head trauma or surgery, eye strain, sinus problems, dental problems, difficulties with opening and closing of the jaw, and the use of medications).
- In office examination (neurological examination; ruling out organic disorders such as aneurysm, stroke, or brain tumor; cluster headachess, trigeminal neuralgia, etc.).
- Laboratory tests (ESR, CBC, blood chemistry to rule out anemia, thyroid disorders, blood and urine culture to rule out infections).

- Other helpful tests: Electroencephalogram (EEG), a Computerized Tomographic (CT) scan and/or a Magnetic Resonance Imaging (MRI) scan).

- Spinal tap to evaluate the cerebrospinal fluids (this will be done in the neurologist's office).

- If the practitioner is not able to get these tests done, the patient should be referred for these tests to appropriate specialist or facility.

LOCATION OF PAIN & CORRESPONDING ACUPUNCTURE MERIDIANS

Information on the location of the pain in association with respective acupuncture meridians is very essential to determine an Oriental medical diagnosis and the plan of treatment using Traditional Chinese medicine and NAET®. These meridians are given with illustration in Chapter 4. Please read and familiarize with these corresponding acupuncture meridians to understand your headache.

Back of the head - Bladder meridian

Front of the head (Forehead) - Stomach meridian

Side(s) of the head - Gall bladder meridian

Top of the head - Liver meridian

Eyeball(s) - Stomach and Colon meridians

STANDARD TREATMENT IN GENERAL

There are two kinds of treatment plans for headaches.

Abortive: Abortive treatment is used with headaches that are already in progress. Pharmacuetical support is used if needed.

Prophylactic: Prophylactic treatments are used to prevent headaches from occurring.

The treatment of the headache depends on the type and severity of the headache and on other factors such as the age of the patient.

ALTERNATIVE MEDICAL TREATMENTS

A number of alternative treatments have been used by practitioners and patients to find relief from headaches. These include:

- Acupuncture or Acupressure
- Chiropractic
- NAET® (Nambudripad's Allergy Elimination Treatments)
- Herbal Remedies
- Homeopathic Remedies
- Transcutaneous Electrical Nerve Stimulation
- Massage Therapy
- Trigger Point Therapy
- Mega Vitamins and Mineral Supplements

Many patients find relief from their head pains using various home remedies. Some of the popular ones are:

- Hydrotherapy
- Cold compresses
- Regular physical exercise
- Relaxation techniques, such as meditation and yoga

PROGNOSIS IN GENERAL

As painful as headaches can be, they are not fatal (as long as they are not a symptom of some more serious disease or disorder). They do not have harmful long-term effects except losing workdays and having a poor quality of life. Most primary types headaches get better on their own after certain number of hours or are relieved by the treatments mentioned above. Secondary types of headaches arise from more serious types of causes. They need immediate attention by the respective specialists.

PREVENTION IN GENERAL

- Prevention is the best solution for headaches. You can avoid primary type headaches by determining the triggers and avoiding them. Read Chapter 5 to learn more about the methods to detect your food and other allergies and avoid the allergy triggers. If you know your tension headaches are related to stress, try to avoid or reduce stress in everyday life.

- Regular acupuncture and/or chiropractic treatments to maintain normal nerve energy circulation through the body.

- Try to find an NAET® practitioner near you and eliminate the causes and/or triggers of your headaches via NAET®.

- Maintaining a daily record of your activities can help to track the pattern of your headaches including the number of times and intensity of each attack of all headaches.

- Adopt lifestyle changes such as exercise, meditation, yoga, relaxation techniques, biofeedback, massages, sauna, hot baths, herbs, counseling, physical therapies, changing jobs, changing living environments, eating nonallergic, nutritious foods, etc.

- Avoid all known allergic foods, drinks, fabrics, and other environmental items. Use the techniques described in Chapter 5 to detect your allergies to all items around you.

- Avoid smoking, tobacco, caffeine, and other stimulants

- Reduce physical and emotional stress

- If the headache persists see a neurologist and have all necessary laboratory tests and radiology tests done to rule out other underlying causes.

MIGRAINE HEADACHES

WHAT IS IT?

Migraines are vascular headaches. The dilation and contraction of blood vessels inside the brain, or an inflammatory substance are thought to be the culprit for migraines. In about 20 percent of migraine cases, the headaches are preceded by visual, auditory or physical auras, bright spots or uneven, unstable lines moving before the eyes.

TYPES OF MIGRAINES

CLASSIC MIGRAINE

This is distinguished by a brief period of warning symptoms 10–60 minutes before an acute attack. Aura is a significant feature of classic migraine, which may include such symptoms as seeing flashing lights or zigzag patterns, temporary loss of vision, difficulty speaking, weakness in an arm or leg, and tingling sensations in the face or hands.

COMMON MIGRAINE

This type of migraine is not preceded by an aura. Some patients may suffer from indigestion, nausea, vomiting, loose stools, depression, mood changes, unusual tiredness, frequent urination, or fluid retention shortly before an attack.

OTHER TYPES OF MIGRAINES

HEMIPLEGIC MIGRAINE

This is characterized by temporary paralysis on one side of the body.

OCCULAR MIGRAINE

In this type the pain is felt in the area around the eye.

BASILAR ARTERY MIGRAINE

In this type, the major artery at the base of the brain is involved. Some statistics show that this type mostly affects young women.

HEADACHE-FREE MIGRAINE

The main feature of this type is the gastrointestinal and visual symptoms of classic migraine, but does not involve head pain.

STATISTICS ON MIGRAINES

The most common type of vascular headache is migraine. More than 29.5 million Americans suffer from migraine, with women being affected three times more often than men. Migraine victims alone lose over 94 million workdays each year because of headache. Migraine attacks usually develop between the ages of five and 35 and experienced between the ages of 15 and 55, and 70% to 80% of sufferers have a family history of migraine. Each individual attack usually lasts from four to 72 hours. Less than half of all migraine sufferers have received a diagnosis of migraine from their health care provider. About one in six women have migraine headaches; women experience migraines three times more often than men. A child may have as high as a 50 percent greater chance of developing migraines if one parent suffers from the disease. The odds jump to 75 percent if both parents experience migraines. Migraine is often misdiagnosed as sinus headache or tension-type headache.

POSSIBLE CAUSES OF MIGRAINES

Migraine headaches are thought to occur when blood vessels in the brain dilate. Brain tissue itself does not feel pain, but other kinds of tissue in and around the brain can feel pain. For example, the nerves that supply to the muscles in the scalp, sinuses inside the head, face, neck, shoulders, the blood vessels supply blood to the base of the brain, can get irritated for various reasons (sensitivities to foods, chemicals and environmental factors, etc.) and cause muscular contractions leading to head pains. The nerve irritation can also disturb the blood and lymph circulation preventing proper circulation causing swelling of the affected tissue that will in turn produce pain in the muscles and tissues on the skull.

COMMON TRIGGERS OF MIGRAINES

Many factors can trigger migraine attacks:

• Diet: - food allergies, sensitivities to certain foods such as caffeine, chocolate, red wine, onion, tyramine, aged cheese, salt, spices, sugar, etc.

• Hormone changes or irregularities: - women may experience migraines at certain times in menstrual cycle, ovulatory cycle, when they are taking oral contraceptives, or after menopause. Sometimes women crave different foods like salty, spicy, sour or sweet foods just a couple of days prior to menstrual periods. An allergy to salty or spicy foods causes fluid retention leading to tissue swelling, nerve irritation and pain. If the allergy caused the fluid retention and edema in the tissue above the neck, they may experience headaches prior to periods. It is a known fact that often women gain 5 to 10 pounds before their periods and lose them afterwards. Any water retention, edema and the resulting pain (headaches or backaches) before or during menstrual periods or cycles have been associated with premenstrual syndromes.

- Irregular carbohydrate metabolism: - hypoglycemia or hyperglycemia (missing meals, delayed meals, etc.)

- Stress related: - Inadequate rest, increased stress, or alteration of sleep-wake cycle.

- Thyroid problems: - hypothyroidism or hyperthyroidism

- Drugs related: - allergic reactions to medications used for other reasons.

- Visual disturbances: - visual problems, unsuitable prescription eye glasses, (or an allergy to eye glasses), irregular lighting (Bright lights, flashing lights, sunlight, fluorescent lights, TV and watching movie).

- Psychological issues: - various emotional stressors.

- Weather Changes: wind, rain, cloudiness, pollen, extreme heat or cold, etc.

- Abnormal sensory Functions: - smells of perfume, cooking smells, any strong odors from surroundings; excessive noise from airplanes, etc.

- Allergy to people, animals or other environmental factors.

SYMPTOMS OF MIGRAINES

Migraine headaches are characterized by throbbing or pulsating pain of moderate or severe intensity lasting from four hours to as long as three days or more. The pain is typically felt on one side of the head: in fact, the English word "migraine" is a combination of two Greek words that mean "half" and "head." Migraine headaches become worse with physical activity.

Migraine characteristics can include pain on one side of the head only (most of the time), pain may be with pulsating or throbbing nature, unable to continue daily activities as usual, may be accompanied by nausea or vomiting, attacks may last for 72 hours or longer, visual disturbances may occur and patient may see aura, and usually exertion makes the headache worse. Some children may get abdominal migraines - A type of migraine that mainly occurs in childhood, characterized by abdominal pain, nausea, vomiting, and sometimes diarrhea, but with little or no headache. Later in life, children with abdominal migraine may develop more typical migraine attacks.

DIAGNOSIS OF MIGRAINES

A detailed medical history should be the first step to diagnose any medical disorders. The history should include past head trauma or surgery, eye strain, sinus problems, dental problems, difficulties with opening and closing of the jaw, and the use of medications. The patient and/or the care taker should cooperate to provide complete medical history to the doctor.

Your doctor then would perform a thorough in office examination to rule out organic disorders such as aneurysm, stroke, or brain tumor; cluster headachess, trigeminal neuralgia, etc.

Laboratory tests (complete blood count, blood chemistry and thyroid profile) will be done to rule out anemia, infections or thyroid disorders, etc. Other useful laboratory tests would be Immunoglobulin studies for specific antigen(s) to detect any involvement with food allergies.

Radiological scans and tests such as electroencephalogram (EEG), a computed tomographic (CT) scan and/or a magnetic resonance imaging (MRI) scan) are useful to confirm presence or absence of any organic causes for the headaches.

Usually, the physical examination of a patient with migraine headache in between the attacks of migraine does not reveal any organic causes for the headaches. Currently there are no definite tests to confirm the diagnosis of migraine.

Information on the location of the pain in association with respective acupuncture meridians is very essential to make a diagnosis of headache using Oriental medical theory and procedures. the location of the headache is very important to plan effective treatment using NAET®.

STANDARD TREATMENT FOR MIGRAINES

Throughout history, many methods have been used to treat migraines. Drilling holes in the skull (Trepanation) was at one time considered to be standard treatment especially for migraines. Ancient Romans found some results to control migraines by placing a black torpedo fish on their foreheads, thinking that the electrical shock it produced would cure their migraine. From this derived the idea of treating migraines with electrical or electromagnetic therapies, Occipital Nerve Stimulation (ONS) and Transcranial Magnetic Stimulation (TMS). A few people find relief with these therapies.

There are two kinds of headache treatment, called abortive and prophylactic. Abortive treatment is used with headaches that are already in progress. Prophylactic treatments are used to prevent headaches from occurring. The treatment of the headache depends on the type and severity of the headache and on other factors such as the age of the patient. Pharmacuetical support

(Amitriptlyine) is often effective if it is taken immediately at the first sign of a migraine.

ALTERNATIVE TREATMENTS FOR MIGRAINES

A number of alternative treatments have been used by practitioners and patients to find relief from headaches. These include:

- Acupuncture or Acupressure
- Chiropractic
- NAET® (Nambudripad's Allergy Elimination Treatments)
- Herbal Remedies
- Homeopathic Remedies
- Transcutaneous Electrical Nerve Stimulation
- Massage Therapy
- Trigger Point Therapy
- Mega Vitamins and Mineral Supplements

Many patients find relief from their head pains using various home remedies. Some of the popular ones are:

- Hydrotherapy
- Cold compresses
- Regular physical exercise
- Relaxation techniques, such as meditation and yoga

PROGNOSIS OF MIGRAINES

Most headaches disappear when the triggers are detected and removed. The headaches are also relieved by the treatments mentioned above. People suffering from acute or chronic migraines can get full freedom from their headaches when they go through a series of NAET®. The NAET® procedures can detect and eliminate most migraine triggers.

PREVENTION OF MIGRAINES

People can avoid migraines by avoiding the factors that trigger them. For example, headaches caused by food allergies can be prevented by not eating the foods that bring on the headaches. One should keep good track of daily activities and a list of foods taken in a diary so that detecting the triggers will be easy. Now you can find out your migraine triggers using NAET testing procedures described in Chapter 5.

Find an NAET® practitioner and eliminate the causes and/or triggers of your migraines via effective NAET®.

Please visit www.naet.com to locate a well trained NAET® practitioner near you.

TENSION HEADACHE

WHAT IS IT?

This is the most common type of headache in the general population. It is also called cephalalgia or muscle contraction headache. It is estimated that more than three-quarters of all headaches are tension-type headaches or triggered by musculo-skeletal causes. The usual tension headache is described as a tightening around the head and neck, accompanied by a steady ache that forms a tight band around the forehead.

TYPES OF TENSION HEADACHE

The International Headache Society classifies tension headaches as either episodic or chronic types.

EPISODIC TENSION HEADACHES

Episodic tension headaches - can occur twice per week but 15 or fewer times per month, whereas chronic tension headaches occur more than 15 times per month when we observe over a period of six months or longer.

CHRONIC TENSION HEADACHES

Chronic tension headaches - can occur daily, bilateral location, usually occipitofrontal and associated with contracted muscles of the neck and scalp. According to International Headache Society, chronic Tension-Type Headaches can strike more than 15 times per month.

STATISTICS ON TENSION HEADACHES

Tension headache can be severe but felt for a short period of time, often a few minutes to a few hours. According to the statistics, about 82% resolve in less than a day. According to researchers, tension-type headaches have not been linked to hereditary factors, even though, 40 percent have family history of headache. Usually, tension headache begins after the age of 50, but 60% have the first onset after 20 years of age. It is predominant more in females than males.

POSSIBLE CAUSES OF TENSION HEADACHES

Both types of tension headaches may be caused by some stressful events. The stressful events trigger muscular contractions and tightening of the muscles in the neck or upper back region. Tension headaches typically result from tightening of these muscles of the face, neck, scalp and also as a result of emotional stress; physical stress (wrong position of the neck and /or shoulder, living near an allergic object like crystal or a piece of furniture, etc.), physiological stress (depression or anxiety); structural stress that force the head and neck muscles to tense (while working in front of a computer, or holding a phone against the ear with one's shoulder); temporomandibular joint dysfunction (TMJ); torticollis, and/ or degenerative arthritis of the neck. The tense muscles put pressure on the nerves that supply the neck, upper back or shoulders and irritate the corresponding nerves and nerve roots. The message of irritation is communicated to the brain via the efferent and afferent nerve fibers through spinal tract. This in turn activates the pain fibers supplying to the affected area and the pain is continued until it is turned off by some means or the person physically moves away from the original source of the stress. When the person continues to live near the object that is causing sensitivity reaction or live without removing the original stress, the headache continues without responding to the prescription medication, or pain relieving therapies. The headache usually disappears after the stress is over.

COMMON TRIGGERS OF TENSION HEADACHES

Tension headaches are thought to be caused when muscles in and around the head contract (tighten up) due to stress or poor posture. Tension headaches are also triggered by eye-strain, over-exertion, loud noises, and allergies or sensitivities to the environmental factors.

- Poor posture

- Stress and/or anxiety

- Depression (found in 70% of those with daily headache)

- Low serotonin level

- Cervical osteoarthritis

- Intramuscular vasoconstriction

- Temporomandibular Joint Syndrome (TMJ)

- Dental alignment problems

- Allergies

SYMPTOMS OF TENSION HEADACHES

Musculoskeletal system is affected in tension headaches. Usually, physical activity does not aggravates tension headache. They are not associated with nausea, vomiting, abdominal pain, weakness or numbness on any one side of the body. They do not usually accompany any visual disturbances, increased sensitivity around light, sound, or difficulty in speaking (slurred speech). But a few people may suffer from a combination of tension headache and migraine headache both at the same time. In such people the symptoms may overlap.

In the case of an acute type of tension headache, the patient will usually describe the pain of a tension headache as mild to moderate in intensity. The severity of the pain varies from one person to another, and from one headache to another in the same person. Most people report that the pain starts soon after waking in the morning, especially if they had an allergy to something in the bed such as pillow, detergent used on the bedsheet or the pillow case, or slept in a wrong position for long hours or slept under a full blowing ceiling fan without proper clothes causing the exposed nerves to contract due to cold air directly affecting them. In the course of a general physical or neurological examination, usually the doctor may not find anything abnormal. Many tense areas, sore spots and trigger points may be felt by the examiner. The trigger points are usually felt on sides of the forehead, around the eyes, top of the head, upper back, neck and paraspinal muscles of the cervical vertebrae, upper part of the shoulder and in the upper trapezius muscles (on one side or both sides).

A chronic type of tension headache usually affects both sides of the head and usually appear at the front of the head, although they can appear at the top or back of the skull. This type of tension headache often begins in the afternoon and can last for several hours. They can occur every day. In some cases, chronic muscle-contraction headaches can last for weeks, months, and sometimes years resulting in insomnia, fatigue, irritability, poor appetite, poor concentration, lack of interest in daily activities and socialization.

DIAGNOSIS OF TENSION HEADACHES

A detailed medical history (should include past head trauma or surgery, eye strain, sinus problems, dental problems, difficulties with opening and closing of the jaw, and the use of medications).

In office examination (neurological examination; ruling out organic disorders such as aneurysm, stroke, or brain tumor; cluster headachess, trigeminal neuralgia, etc.).

Laboratory tests (ESR, CBC, blood chemistry to rule out anemia, infections or thyroid disorders).

Other helpful tests: Electroencephalogram (EEG), a computed tomographic (CT) scan and/or a magnetic resonance imaging (MRI) scan)

If the practitioner is not able to get these tests done, the patient should be referred for these tests to appropriate specialist or facility.

Tests such as the CT scan and MRI are useful to confirm the lack of organic causes for the headaches. Currently there is no definite test to confirm the diagnosis of tension headaches.

Information on the location of the pain in association with respective acupuncture meridians is very essential to determine the plan of treatment in Oriental medicine and with NAET®.

STANDARD TREATMENTS FOR TENSION HEADACHES

These types of headaches usually can be relieved with hot packs over the neck and back muscles, ultra sound massage therapy, trigger point therapy, relaxation exercises, by general relaxation, with over the counter or prescription pain medications, muscle relaxants and especially if one can trace and avoid the stress inducing factor.

ALTERNATIVE TREATMENTS FOR TENSION HEADACHES

A number of alternative treatments have been found effective in helping with tension headaches. These include:

- Acupuncture or acupressure

- Chiropractic

- Herbal remedies

- Homeopathic remedies

- Cold or hot compresses

- Massage and trigger point therapy

- Mega vitamins and mineral supplements

- Regular physical exercise

- Relaxation techniques, such as meditation and yoga

- NAET® (Nambudripad's Allergy Elimination Treatments).

Read Chapter 5 to learn self testing procedures to detect the causative agent for your headaches. Once you find the causative factor, you have two choices: either avoid the causative factor (allergen) or locate a well trained NAET® practitioner from our website (www.naet.com) and eliminate the cause from your life so that you will lead a tension-headache free life for the rest of your life as thousands of people are doing already.

PROGNOSIS OF TENSION HEADACHES

Tension headaches disappear when the triggers are detected and removed. They are also relieved by the treatments mentioned above. People suffering from acute or chronic headaches can get full freedom from their tension headaches when they go through a series of NAET® to detect and eliminate the triggers.

PREVENTION OF TENSION HEADACHES

People can avoid tension headaches by avoiding the factors that trigger them. For example, headaches caused by wearing dry cleaned clothes can be prevented by not getting them cleaned by that method. One should maintain a list of daily activities and a list of items used during the course of any day so that one could locate the triggers easily.

Avoidance of identifiable trigger factors

Healthful life-styles including regular exercise and good eating habits

Reduce physical and emotional stress

Include relaxation techniques and procedures such as biofeedback, acupuncture, chiropractic, massages, sauna, hot baths, herbs, relaxation, yoga, physical therapies, counseling, changing jobs, changing living environments, etc. in your routine activity list.

Find an NAET® practitioner near you and eliminate the causes and/or triggers of your tension headaches via effective NAET®.

Please visit **www.naet.com** to locate a well trained NAET® practitioner near you.

CLUSTER HEADACHES

WHAT IS IT?

Cluster headaches are recurrent brief attacks of sudden and severe pain on one side of the head, similar to migraine and characterized by severe pain in the eye or temple on one side of the head, watering of the eye, and a runny nose and usually most intense pain is in the area around the eye. Cluster headaches may last between five minutes and three hours; they may occur once every other day or as often as eight times per day. This is a form of neurovascular headache, which causes repeated episodes of intense pain, and headaches over weeks or months usually at the same time of day or night. The headaches often occur in clusters, beginning as a minor pain around one eye, eventually spreading to that side of the face. Each headache is brief in duration, typically lasting a few moments to 2 hours. Cluster refers to a grouping of headaches, usually over a period of several weeks. The pain can also become excruciating without warning, causing the person to lose balance, fall on the floor, press hard at the site of pain or bang the head intentionally on a hard surface (wall, floor, etc.) or screaming, seeking some relief. The other names for this type of headaches are histamine headache, Horton neuralgia, or erythromelalgia.

TYPES OF CLUSTER HEADACHES

The International Headache Society has classified cluster headaches as either episodic or chronic cluster headaches. Other types which may be included under the same category are toxic headaches, hypertensive headaches and rebound headaches

EPISODIC CLUSTER HEADACHES

Episodic cluster headaches occur over periods lasting from seven days to one year, with the clusters separated by headache-free intervals of at least two weeks. The average length of a cluster ranges between two weeks and three months.

CHRONIC CLUSTER HEADACHES

In this type, the cluster-free interval is less than 1 week in a 12-month period. About 10 percent to 20 percent of people with cluster headache have the chronic type. Chronic cluster headache may develop after a period of episodic attacks, or it may develop spontaneously, without a prior history of headaches. Some people experience alternating episodic and chronic phases.

OTHER TYPES OF CLUSTER HEADACHES

TOXIC HEADACHES

People get headaches from various circulating toxins in the body due to certain infections. Infections may be primary as in the cases of upper respiratory infections, pneumonia, measles, mumps, infections from ear, nose, and throat causes. Infections may also be due to secondary causes: immunization reaction, vaccination reaction, or as an after effect of certain allergic reactions. Toxic headaches can result from exposures to household chemicals, pesticides, insecticides, dry cleaning agents, mercury, lead, food additives (sulfites, nitrites, monosodium glutamate, meat tenderizer), food flavorings, food colorings, artificial sweeteners, pollution from the atmosphere, toxins from work materials, etc. Toxic reactions to prescription drugs are also very common.

HYPERTENSIVE HEADACHES

Often, headache is present in people who suffer from high blood pressure associated with hypertensive encephalopathy. Headache is the prime manifestation of increased intracranial pressure. High blood pressure can cause headache, but in general is not the cause of recurring headaches. Blood pressure usually has to be quite elevated to cause headache. Allergic reactions to the antihypertensive drugs cause headaches in the people with sensitivity to the very drug that is supposed to help control their hypertension. Patient may present with severe headaches, nausea, and vomiting. On questioning you may discover that the patient stopped taking the blood pressure medication because the patient thought that he/she did not need it anymore.

REBOUND HEADACHES

Rebound headaches happen in people who overuse substances like food, pain killers, and caffeine. People use the pain killers and caffeine products probably to reduce or control headaches. Due to their allergies to the pain killers or caffeine, the products do not help them to reduce headaches always. They begin to consume the products in larger quantities hoping to get relief, eventually they become depended on them. So they take the products to reduce headaches; temporarily they may get relief for a few minutes, then the headaches returns with more intensity, so they double up on the pain killers, then after a few minutes, they get worse headaches. The pain-drug-pain-cycle goes on without getting complete relief. People who have **rebound headaches** also may have nausea, anxiety, irritability, depression, or problems sleeping.

STATISTICS ON CLUSTER HEADACHES

Cluster headaches are more common in men. Cluster headaches usually begin in middle adult life. Mean age of onset is 30 years for men and later for women. Approximately 80 percent of cluster headaches are episodic, that is, they occur during one to five month periods followed by six to twenty-four month attack-free periods . Cluster headaches last between 30 and 45 minutes. Many people have cluster bouts during the spring and fall.

POSSIBLE CAUSES OF CLUSTER HEADACHES

Cluster headaches seem to be associated with alcohol, drugs, tobacco smoke, previous head trauma, tension of the upper back muscles, allergies such as food, drinks, drugs, furniture, pillow, toys, plastics, computer keyboard, TV monitor remote controller, seasonal allergies, etc. Rapid rise in blood pressure due to anger, vigorous exercise, or sexual excitement can also trigger headaches.

SYMPTOMS OF CLUSTER HEADACHES

The pain of a cluster headache is excruciating; some patients describe it as severe enough to make them consider suicide. Patients with cluster headaches are restless; they may pace the floor, weep, rock back and forth, or bang their heads against a wall in desperation to stop the pain. In addition to severe pain, patients with cluster headaches often have various signs of allergies such as a runny or congested nose, watery or inflamed eyes, drooping eyelids, swelling in the area of the eyebrows, and heavy facial perspiration. Most people with a cluster headache prefer to be alone. They may remain outdoors, even in freezing weather, for the duration of an attack. They may scream, bang their heads against a wall or hurt themselves in some way as a distraction from the unbearable pain. Some may find relief by exercising, such as jogging in place or doing sit-ups or push-ups. If cluster headache attacks regularly occur at night the person may also suffer from insomnia. Lack of proper sleep or rest can lead them to depression and thoughts of suicide.

DIAGNOSIS OF CLUSTER HEADACHES

• A detailed medical history (should include past head trauma or surgery, eye strain, sinus problems, dental problems, difficulties with opening and closing of the jaw, and the use of illicit drugs or prescription medications for other conditions).

- In office examination to rule out organic disorders such as aneurysm, stroke, or brain tumor or trigeminal neuralgia, etc.).

- Laboratory tests to rule out anemia, infections or thyroid disorders.

Other Tests: Electroencephalogram (EEG), a computed tomographic (CT) scan and/or a magnetic resonance imaging (MRI) scan)

If the practitioner is not able to get these tests done, the patient should be referred for these tests to appropriate specialist or facility.

Information on the location of the pain in association with respective acupuncture meridians is very essential to determine the plan of treatment using Oriental medicine and NAET®.

Locate the causative agent and eliminate it or avoid it. Stress factor may be different in each person.

STANDARD TREATMENTS FOR CLUSTER HEADACHES

These types of headaches can only be relieved by removing the causative factor from the person's life or surroundings. In the case of drug allergy, sometimes changing drugs may help solve the problem if the patient is not allergic to new drug or substitute.

ALTERNATIVE TREATMENTS FOR CLUSTER HEADACHES

A number of alternative treatments have been recommended for treating and preventing headaches. These include:

- Acupuncture or acupressure

- Chiropractic

- Herbal remedies

- Homeopathic remedies

- Hydrotherapy

- Massage and trigger point therapy

- Mega vitamin and mineral supplements

- Regular physical exercise

- Relaxation techniques, such as meditation and yoga

- NAET® (Nambudripad's Allergy Elimination Treatments).

Use NAET® procedures (Chapter 5) to detect the causative agent for your headaches. Once you find the causative factor, you have two choices: either avoid the causative factor (allergen) or locate a well trained NAET® practitioner and eliminate the cause from your life so that you will lead a cluster-headache free life for rest of your life as thousands of people are doing already.

PROGNOSIS OF CLUSTER HEADACHES

Most headaches disappear when the triggers are detected and removed. They are also relieved by the treatments mentioned above. People suffering from acute or chronic migraines can get full freedom from their headaches when they go through a series of NAET® to detect and eliminate their triggers.

PREVENTION OF CLUSTER HEADACHES

People can avoid some headaches by avoiding the factors that trigger them. For example, headaches caused by food allergies can be prevented by not eating the foods that bring on the headaches. One should keep good track of daily activities and a list of foods taken in a diary so that detecting the triggers will be easy.

Avoidance of identifiable trigger factors

Healthful life-styles including regular exercise and good eating habits

Avoid allergic foods or drinks

Avoid smoking, tobacco, caffeine, and other stimulants

Reduce physical and emotional stress

Encourage the use of non-pharmacological techniques to control or reduce headaches such as: biofeedback, acupuncture, chiropractic, massages, sauna, hot baths, herbs, relaxation, yoga, physical therapies, counseling, changing jobs, changing living environments, etc.

Find an NAET® practitioner and eliminate the causes and/or triggers of your cluster headaches via effective NAET®.

Please visit **www.naet.com** to locate a well trained NAET® practitioner near you.

SECONDARY HEADACHES

TRACTION HEADACHES

Traction headaches are serious, pathologic headaches caused by tumors, cysts, aneurysms or other changes within the brain. Traction headaches result from the pulling, stretching, or displacing of structures that are sensitive to pain, as when a brain tumor presses on the outer layer of nerve tissue that covers the brain. Traction headaches are warning for more serious problems. These may be arising from traction on intracranial structures, mainly by masses, metastatic tumors, hematomas, abscesses, post-lumbar puncture headaches that do not stop after a few hours, chronic intracranial pressure due to unknown reasons. They should be brought to the attention of the appropriate specialist without delay.

HEADACHES DUE TO BRAIN TUMORS

Headaches associated with brain tumors usually begin as episodic nighttime headaches that are accompanied by projectile vomiting. The headaches may become continuous over time, and usually get worse if the patient coughs, sneezes, bears down while using the toilet, or does something else that increases the pressure inside the head.

HEADACHES DUE TO MENINGITIS

Toxins produced by bacteria or virus begin to overload and circulate in the body leading to energy disturbances in the energy supply to the various parts of the brain leading to intermittent or continuous severe headaches, high fever, and photophobia. Headaches may continue chronically until the infection is resolved.

HEAD INJURY CAUSING HEADACHES

Patients may complain of headaches as well as poor memory, lack of concentration, general irritability, restlessness, irregular sleep pattern, and general fatigue for months or even years after a head injury. These symptoms are known as post-concussion syndrome. In some cases, a blow on the head may cause some blood vessels to rupture and produce a hematoma, or mass of blood that displaces brain tissue, and can cause seizures as well as headaches.

HEADACHES RESULTING FROM SPINAL PROCEDURES

About 25% of patients who undergo a lumbar puncture (spinal tap) for diagnostic purpose or therapeutic purpose (spinal anaesthesia, etc.) may develop a headache from the lowered cerebrospinal fluid pressure around the brain and spinal cord. Lumbar puncture headaches usually go away on their own after a few hours.

REFERRED HEADACHES

This type of pain is felt in a part of the body at a distance from the injured or diseased area. Headache pain may be referred from diseased teeth; disks in the cervical spine that have been damaged by spondylosis (degeneration of the spinal vertebrae caused by osteoarthritis); or the temporomandibular joint, the small joint in front of the ear where the lower jaw is attached to the skull.

IDIOPATHIC INTRACRANIAL PRESSURE TRIGGERING HEADACHES

Increased pressure inside the skull in the absence of any abnormality of the central nervous system or blockage in the flow of the cerebrospinal fluid has been found to be a trigger for headaches. After careful examination, some allergic factor may be seen as the cause for increased intracranial pressure. In addition to headache, patients with this disorder experience diplopia (seeing double) and other visual symptoms.

INFLAMMATORY HEADACHES

Inflammatory headaches are symptoms of other disorders, ranging from stroke to sinus infection. Like other types of pain, headaches can serve as warning signals of more serious disorders. This is particularly true for headaches caused by inflammation, including those related to meningitis, temporal arteritis, trigeminal neuralgia, as well as those resulting from diseases of the sinuses, spine, neck, ears, and teeth. Headache that is a symptom of another disorder, such as sinus infection. Trauma, exertion, rebound headaches, dental work related and temporomandibular joint related headaches, foods, chemical, environmental sensitivities and allergies triggered headaches and organic causes fall in this category.

HEADACHES TRIGGERED BY SINUS INFECTIONS

Facial and head pain resulting from sinusitis is considered an inflammatory headache. Acute sinusitis is characterized by fluid buildup inside sinus cavities inflamed by a bacterial or viral infection. Chronic sinusitis usually results from an allergic reaction to smoke, dust, animal fur, or similar irritants. Headache and pain related to sinusitis are referred pains resulting from stimulation of the sensory nerves that supply the sinus cavities. Stimulation of these nerves occurs in response to a diseased sinus. The most common is stimulation associated with sinusitis. Each of us has four paired cavities in our head that communicate with the nose through narrow channels. These cavities produce a thick mucus that drains out of the channels into the nose. A cold or flu might cause swelling in these narrow channels, preventing the outflow of mucus. When this happens, bacteria might grow in the closed space of the sinus and cause an infection, leading to sinus headaches.

HEADACHES TRIGGERED BY TEMPORAL ARTERITIS

Temporal arteritis is an inflammation of the temporal artery that most commonly affects people over 50. In addition to headache, patients with temporal arteritis may have fever, loss of appetite, and blurring or loss of vision and pain in the jaw during mastication. Food allergies may cause the inflammation.

HEADACHES BEFORE OR AFTER STROKE

Headaches may be associated with several conditions that may lead to stroke, including high blood pressure and heart disease. Headaches may also result from completed stroke or from the mini-strokes known as transient ischemic attacks, or TIAs.

Find an NAET® practitioner near you and have an NAET evaluation of your headache by him or her. NAET treatments are often able to help with your symptoms temporarily and provide you with symptomatic relief even if they are arising from organic causes. NAET does not interfere with any other treatment you are getting. In fact NAET can enhance the treatment effect of other procedures by assisting to eliminate any possible allergic factors or emotional fear about the condition involved with your health condition.

Please visit **www.naet.com** to locate a well trained NAET® practitioner near you.

WHEN YOU SHOULD SEEK MEDICAL HELP?

Not all headaches require immediate medical attention. Some result from hypoglycemia, muscle tension, and common cold or flu triggered headaches. These can be easily controlled using over the counter medications, decongestants, home remedies or any available alternative therapies. But some types of headache are warning signs of more serious disorders, and call for prompt medical care. These include:

- Sudden, severe headache

- Sudden, severe headache associated with a stiff neck

- Headache associated with fever

- Headache associated with convulsions

- Headache accompanied by confusion or loss of consciousness

- Headache following a blow on the head

- Headache associated with pain in the eye or ear

- Persistent headache in a person who was previously headache free

- Recurring headache in children

- Headache that interfere with normal life

WHAT IS NAET®?

NAET® is a non-invasive, drug free, natural solution to eliminate allergies and energy disturbances of all types and intensities using a blend of selective energy balancing, testing and treatment procedures from acupuncture/acupressure, allopathy, chiropractic, Kinesiology, and nutritional disciplines of medicine.

THE BASIS OF NAET®

A thorough treatise on biochemistry is not appropriate for an introduction to this new method of treatment for people suffering from allergies. Instead, this discussion will concentrate on the basic constructs of the treatment method and give some insight into the lives of the people it has helped.

This is not a new technology. It is actually a combination of knowledge and techniques that uses much of what is already known from allopathic (Western medical knowledge), chiropractic, kinesiology, acupuncture (Oriental medical knowledge) and nutrition. Each of the disciplines I studied provided bits of knowledge which I used in developing this new treatment.

Until now, there has been no known permanent successful method of treatment for headaches using Western medicine except controlling the symptoms using drugs.

I have developed this treatment for headaches using Nambudripad's allergy elimination techniques or NAET® because in most cases of headaches whether it may be migraines, tension headaches or cluster headaches if we search carefully, always we can find an allergic involvement: an allergy to a food eaten just before the headache began or came in contact with a chemical or exposed to an environmental allergen or may be an emotionally upsetting event.

HOW WAS NAET® DISCOVERED?

NAET® was discovered by an accident on Friday, November 23, 1983, at about 2:00 PM. I was being treated by acupuncture for the relief of a severe allergic reaction to raw carrots. During the treatment, I fell asleep with the carrots still in my hand on my body. After the acupuncture treatment (and a restful nap during the needling period), I woke up and experienced a unique sense of well-being. I had never felt quite that way following other similar acupuncture treatments in the past. I realized that I had been lying on some of the carrot pieces. A piece was also still in my hand. I knew that some of the needles were supposed to help circulate the electrical energy and balance the body. If there is any energy blockage, the balancing process is supposed to clear it during the treatment and bring the body to a balanced state. I had studied this concept in school.

I asked my husband, who was assisting me in the treatment process, to test me for carrots again using NST (Neuromuscular

Sensitivity Testing explained in detail in Chapter 5). After putting "two and two together," I understood that the carrot's energy field had interacted with my own energy field, and my brain had accepted this once deadly poison to my body as a harmless item now after balancing the two energies during the acupuncture treatment. The two energy fields no longer clashed. This was an amazing NEW DISCOVERY. Subsequent tests for carrots by NST confirmed that something phenomenal had happened. We repeated testing every hour for the rest of that day. I continued eating carrots the next day without any allergic reaction. This confirmed the result. My central nervous system had learned a different response to the stimulus arriving from carrot and I was no longer reactive to it. In some mysterious way, the treatment had reprogrammed my brain.

What followed was a series of experiments treating my own allergies and those of my family. I cleared most of my allergies in a year's time. The method was eventually extended to my practice. In every case, allergies were "cleared out," never to return.

After having treated thousands of patients for a wide variety of allergens, the procedure is no longer experimental or of questionable value. It is a proven treatment method and the premise of NAET® methodology that is now being followed by more than 9,000 health care professionals around the world.

During my practice I saw numerous patients who suffered from cephalalgia and various types of headaches. I treated them with traditional chiropractic, a few with acupuncture and herbs but I offered a few patients NAET treatments and they were happy to receive those free treatments. The patients who were treated with NAET got complete relief from their headaches without any drugs or therapies. Soon the word spread among their friends and families, patients with various types of headaches became the major part of my practice. Usually patients who are reluctant to take drugs go to chiropractors or acupuncturists. Since I was a chiropractor and an acupuncturist, people with different types of headaches found comfort in my office. When we did a ten-year survey of our treatment records it was shown that over a period of ten years we treated 1849 headache patients (1243 patients with general headaches (tension, cluster, etc.) and 606 patients with migraines) in our office with NAET®, Out of 1,849 patients treated 21 patients were referred out to other specialists for further treatments. Rest of the patients resolved their headaches in our office with NAET®.

OVERVIEW OF NAET®

Physical contact with the allergen during and after a treatment (which consists of stimulating certain specific points on the acupuncture meridians, thus stimulating the central nervous system) produces the necessary immune mediators or antidotes to neutralize the adverse reaction coming from the allergen held in the hand. This produces a totally new, permanent and irreversible response to the allergen. It is possible, through stimulation of the appropriate points of the acupuncture meridians, (which have direct correspondence with the brain), to reprogram the brain.

A living person's body is made up of bones, flesh, lymph, nerves and blood vessels, which can only function in the presence of vital energy. Like electricity, vital energy is not visible to the human eye.

No one knows how the vital energy gets into the body or how, when or where it goes when it leaves. It is true, however, that without it, none of the body functions can take place. When the body is alive, vital energy flows freely through the energy pathways. Uninterrupted circulation of the vital energy flowing through the energy pathways is necessary to keep the person alive and healthy. This circulation of energy makes all the body functions possible. The circulation of the vital energy makes the blood travel through the blood vessels, helping to distribute appropriate nutrients to various parts of the body for its growth, development, functions, and for repair of wear and tear.

The success of the NAET® procedure confirms that a major portion of the illnesses we observe result from allergies. Headaches are not any different from other diseases.

The public should be educated to find the cause of the problems. If the cause can be traced, you can easily avoid contact with the causative agent. If contact is unavoidable, you can go to any of the nine thousand plus NAET® trained medical professionals who have mastered the NAET® method of eliminating the root cause of the health disorders - an allergy to something somewhere - so that you don't have to avoid the item for ever.

NAET® has its origin in Oriental medicine. If one explores most Oriental medical books–acupuncture textbooks, one may not find the NAET® interpretation of health problems that I write in my books, because NAET® is my sole development after observing my own reactions, my family's and patients' over the past two decades. Recently, however, information about the effectiveness of NAET® has been given credit in a number of books, but the reader will find correct information of NAET® interpretation of Oriental medical principles only in my books.

In this book, information about acupuncture meridians is kept to a minimum, enough to educate the reader about some traditional functions and dysfunctions of the meridians in the presence of energy disturbances. Some of this information is also available in acupuncture textbooks that one may find in libraries. It is a good idea to have some understanding of Oriental medicine and the meridians when undergoing NAET® treatments although it is not mandatory. To learn more about acupuncture meridians and mindbody connections, please read Chapter 10 in my book Say Goodbye to Illness.

Say Good-bye to Headaches

NAET® utilizes a variety of standard medical procedures to diagnose and then treat allergies and allergy-related health conditions. These include: standard medical diagnostic procedures and standard allergy testing procedures (read Chapter 3). After detecting allergies, NAET® uses standard chiropractic and acupuncture/acupressure procedures to eliminate them. Various studies have proven that NAET® is capable of erasing the previously encoded incorrect message about an allergen and replacing it with a harmless or useful message by reprogramming the brain. (Please read the Journal of NAET® Energetics and Complementary Medicine, Vol 1, 2, 3 and 4, 2005; Vol 5, 6, 7 and 8, 2006.) This is accomplished by bringing the body into a state of "homeostasis" using various NAET® energy balancing techniques.

Chiropractic theory postulates that a pinching of the spinal nerve root(s) may cause nerve energy disturbance in the energy pathways causing poor nerve energy supply to the target organs (disturbance in the functions of afferent and efferent nerves). When the particular nerve fails to communicate with a particular area of the organs and tissues, normal functions of that area do not take place. The affected organs and tissues then begin to manifest impaired functions in digestion, absorption, assimilation and elimination.

In chiropractic theory, an allergy can be seen as a result of a pinched nerve. Impaired functions of the organs and tissues will improve when the pinching of the spinal nerves is removed (by removing the disturbances in the afferent and efferent nerve functions) and energy circulation is restored through chiropractic adjustments. But the adjustments have to be applied on a regular basis. Otherwise the misalignment could return. I believe that an allergic reaction initiates the pinching of the spinal nerve root resulting in reduced nerve energy supply to the target-tissues and/or organ. The poor energy supply will lead to poor blood supply to the target tissue. Poor blood supply will lead to reduced nutrients and oxygen supply to the specific area. The organs and tissues need

48

uninterrupted supply of oxygen and nutrients through days and nights for their normal function. When there is a disturbance in this energy supply, the area will begin to send warning signs to the brain and these warning signs will manifest as aches and pains. If the tissue on the head was the said target tissue, then the aches and pains will be felt on various parts of the head and we call that pain as headaches. When the allergen is located through NST (Neuromuscular Sensitivity Testing), when it is desensitized through NAET, pinching of the nerve root will be stopped thus restoring the nerve energy flow to the target organs and tissues. This will in turn eliminate the headaches.

I observed my regular chiropractic patients for a long time. I did not have an explanation for the need for "the twice a week" regular chiropractic treatment to keep the body in alignment. Then I combined NAET® with regular chiropractic treatment. When these patients began desensitization for the NAET® basic essential nutrients (NAET® Basic allergens) through NAET®, we noticed that they were holding adjustments for longer times. By the time they completed desensitization on 25 to 30 NAET Basic allergen groups, most of these patients responded very well health-wise. Their aches and pains were reduced, headaches were minimized, backaches were almost gone in most cases and other symptoms also reduced greatly. They digested their meals better. Sleep improved. Overall energy increased many fold. The quality of life improved. They maintained their spinal alignments without losing them so they did not need frequent chiropractic adjustments as before. The observation of these patients invoked enough interest to study the benefits of NAET® on a larger group and we received similar results. From this observation I concluded that allergens are the cause of spinal misalignment, pinched nerves and various types of headaches.

Oriental medicine explains the same theory from a different perspective. In Oriental medicine, the balance of Yin and Yang represents the perfect balance of energies (the state of homeostasis). Any interference in the energy flow or an energy disturbance can cause an imbalance in the Yin-Yang state and an imbalance in "homeostasis." Any substance that is capable of creating an energy disturbance in one's body is called an allergen.

According to NAET® theory, when a substance is brought into the electromagnetic field of an individual, an attraction or repulsion takes place between the energy of the individual and the substance.

ATTRACTION BETWEEN ENERGIES

If two energies are attracted to each other, both energies benefit each other. The individual can benefit from association with the substance. The energy of the substance will combine with the energy of the individual and enhance functional ability. For example: After taking an antibiotic, the bacterial infection is diminished. Here the energy of the antibiotic joins forces with the energy of the body and helps to eliminate the bacteria. Another example is taking vitamin supplements (if one is not allergic to them) and the gaining of energy and vitality.

REPULSION BETWEEN ENERGIES

If two energies repel each other, they are not good for each other. The individual can experience the repulsion of his/her energy from the other as a discomfort in the body. The energy of the individual will cause energy blockages in his/her energy meridians to prevent invasion of the adverse energy into his/her energy field. For example: After taking a repelling antibiotic, not only does the bacterial infection not get better but the individual might break out in rashes all over the body causing fever, nausea, excessive perspiration, fatigue, etc. If repulsion takes place between two energies, then the substance that is capable of producing the repulsion in a living individual is considered an allergen. When the allergen produces a repulsion of energy in the electromagnetic field, certain energy disturbance takes place in the body. The energy disturbance caused from the repulsion of the substance is capable of producing various unpleasant or adverse reactions. These reactions are considered "allergic reactions."

NATURAL BODY DEFENSE

In certain instances, the body also produces many natural body defenses like "histamine, immunoglobulins, etc." to help the body overcome the unpleasant reactions from the interaction with the allergen. The most common immunoglobulin produced during a reaction is called IgE (immunoglobulin E). The activation of IgE antibodies causes what the traditional medical profession calls "true" allergies; however, millions of people experience various allergic symptoms every day in varying degrees without producing these antibodies. These types of reactions can be called either intolerance or hypersensitivity.

When the body is exposed to what it thinks is a foreign and dangerous substance, a normal immune system will immediately release chemical mediators appropriate to the condition to counteract the allergic reaction. The body will come to a settlement with the allergen in seconds without causing any obvious ill-health symptoms in the body. But when the immune system perceives what should be harmless substances as dangerous intruders and stimulates antibody production to defend the body, things do not settle down as pleasantly as in the individual with a normal immune system. Here, the first contact with an allergen initiates the baby step of an allergic reaction inside the body. The body will alert its defense forces in response to the alarm received about the new invader and will immediately produce a few antibodies, storing them in reserve for future use.

In most cases, a first contact or initial sensitization will usually not produce many symptoms. During the second exposure to the allergen, the body will alert the previously produced antibodies to action, producing more noticeable symptoms. If you have a strong immune system, the second exposure may not cause too many unpleasant symptoms either. But often, with the third exposure, the threatened immune system will begin serious action by producing massive amounts of antibodies to defend against the invader, causing what the traditional allergist calls an allergic reaction.

Various types of immunoglobulins are produced in the body at various times as natural defense mechanisms to protect the body. They include: IgE, IgA, IgD, IgG, and IgM.

Some people could have only the IgE mediated allergies, in which case IgE antibodies can be found in the blood sample. Some others can have more than one antibody in their blood, depending on how many allergens they have reacted to in the past.

People suffer from various types of headaches (allergic manifestation) in varying degrees because of the above mentioned reasons. Regardless of age, gender, race, or inheritance, anyone can manifest headaches at any time if the circumstances fall within the above causes.

In sensitive individuals, contact with any allergen can produce a variety of symptoms, in varying degrees including headaches. The ingested, inhaled or contacted allergens are capable of alerting the body's immune system. The frightened and confused immune system then commands the production and immediate release of immunoglobulins and other chemical mediators.

In order to enjoy life, the patients with headaches must find the causative factors and overcome their adverse reactions to the allergens. It can be done through NAET.

HOME EVALUATION PROCEDURES

Do you suffer from any allergy? Or Allergy-related disorder? Below is an allergy-check list to help you evaluate yourself to see if you have any active or hidden allergies. A sensible solution can be found if you can identify the source of your problem.

1. Please describe your headache in one sentence.

_____

When did your headache begin? Please write approximate date and time if you don't remember the exact date, time and event._____

Rate your symptoms and headache on a scale of 0-10, here "0" equals no symptom or discomfort and "10" equals maximum discomfort.

2. How is your energy at these following hours?

6 am [ ], 8 am [ ], 10 am [ ], 12 noon [ ], 2 PM [ ],

4 PM [ ], 6 PM [ ], 6 PM [ ], 8 PM [ ], 10 PM [ ],

12 am [ ], 2 am [ ], 4 am [ ]

3. How is your appetite? ——————— [ ]

4. How is your digestion? ——————— [ ]

5. How is your elimination? ————————[ ]

6. How is your sleep? ——————— [ ]

7. How is your general well-being? – [ ]

ORGAN-MERIDIAN ASSOCIATION TIME

It takes two hours to circulate energy through one energy meridian. If the energy can travel through the meridians without any obstruction in the flow, you should feel good overall. If there is any energy disturbance in the meridians, it will reflect on your health depending on the meridian(s) affected. If you feel unusual symptoms or illnesses, note the time of the day you felt differently. After you find the time, find the corresponding meridian (s) from the list below.

NAMES OF THE MERIDIANS

Lung (Lu) .... 3-5 am

Large Intestine (LI) .... 5-7 am

Stomach (St) .... 7-9 am

Spleen (Sp) 9-11am

Heart (Ht) ....11-1 pm

Small Intestine - (SI)......1-3 pm

Urinary Bladder (UB)......3-5 pm

Kidney (Ki) ....5-7 pm

Pericardium (PC or CI)....7-9 pm

Triple warmer (TW)..........9-11pm

Gall Bladder (GB)...........11-1 am

Liver (Lv)......................1-3 am

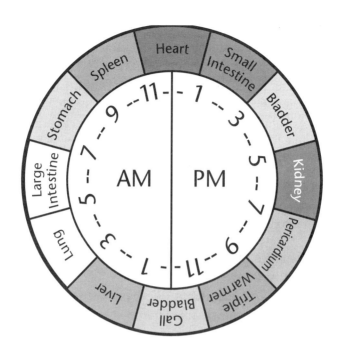

FIGURE 1

ACUPUNCTURE MERIDIAN CLOCK

Say Good-bye to Headaches

Then go to Chapter 4 in this book to find out more about your health. Detailed information about the normal and abnormal functions of the acupuncture meridians is given in Chapter 4. If there is no energy blockage in the meridian(s), then an individual will experience normal functions. In the case of an energy blockage(s), abnormal function(s) can be seen or experienced by the individual. Then go to Chapter 6 to learn the home-balancing techniques. Do it once or twice a day for a few weeks. No matter what condition you are in, your home-balancing treatment will make a difference in your overall health. If the problem is mild you should be able to help eliminate your problem by simply following the home-balancing procedures given in Chapter 6. But if the problem is more than mild, please find a NAET® specialist immediately and have him/her evaluate your condition and do further necessary treatments. We have received numerous testimonials from many users of home-help procedures that by massaging these balancing points on a regular basis, they have been able to get freedom from their headaches.

Please read through the next few pages and evaluate yourself to make a list of possible sensitivities. You will be able to detect most of your sensitivities by yourself if you go through this self-evaluation of your symptoms.

ALLERGY SYMPTOM CHECKLIST

Please read the following list of symptoms in the next few pages. They could be caused from allergies. Many thousands of people have received relief from these symptoms by treating with NAET®. Please rate your symptoms on a scale of 0-3: (0= no symptoms; 1= mild symptoms; 2= moderate symptoms; 3= severe symptoms).

RATING   SYMPTOMS

— Acne

— Addiction to alcohol

— Addiction to caffeine

— Addiction to chocolate

— Addiction to coffee

— Addiction to drugs

— Addiction to food

— Addiction to smoking

— Addiction to sugar

— Addictions to carbohydrate

— Aggression

— Allergy to animals

— Allergy to aspirin

— Allergy to insects

— Allergy to cold

— Allergy to corn

— Allergy to Fish

— Allergy to shellfish

RATING   SYMPTOMS

— Allergy to food additives

— Allergy to food colorings

— Allergy to gasoline

— Allergy to hair dye

— Allergy to heat

— Allergy to humidity

— Allergy to latex

— Allergy to mercury

— Allergy to milk products

— Allergy to mushroom

— Allergy to mold

— Allergy to newspaper ink

— Allergy to nuts

— Allergy to paper

— Allergy to penicillin

— Allergy to perfume

— Allergy to plastics

— Allergy to pollens

— Allergy to proteins

— Allergy to radiation

— Allergy to razor blade

— Allergy to salt

— Allergy to smells

— Allergy to sugar

— Allergy to trees

RATING   SYMPTOMS

— Allergy to weeds

— Allergy to wheat/gluten

— Amnesia temporary

— Anemia

— Angina-like pains

— Anxiety attacks

— Arthritis

— Asthma, bronchial

— Asthma, cardiac

— Athletes foot

— Attention deficit disorder

— Backache

— Bone pains

— Bipolar disorders

— Biting nails

— Blurred vision

— Bowel disorder

— Brain fog

— Breast-pain

— Burning feet

— Burning in the groin

— Burning sensation on urination

— Candida/yeast

— Canker sores

— Cardiac arrhythmia

Chapter 1

RATING   SYMPTOMS

— Cervical dysplasia
— Chronic cough
— Chronic low grade fever
— Chronic nasal congestion
— Clumsiness
— Cold extremities
— Cold intolerance
— Cold sores
— Colitis
— Compulsive behavior
— Constipation
— Craving fat
— Craving spices
— Craving salt
— Craving sour
— Craving sweets
— Craving bitters
— Craving onions
— Crohns' disease
— Conjunctivitis
— Cuts heal slowly
— Dandruff
— Decreased sex drive
— Dermatitis
— Depression

61

RATING   SYMPTOMS

—Diabetes

—Diarrhea

—Difficulty in walking

—Difficulty in swallowing

—Distractibility

— Diverticulitis

—Dizziness

—Dream disturbed sleep

—Dry eyes

—Dry mouth

—Dry skin

—Dryness

—Dyslexia

—Earaches

—Ear infections

—Eating dirt

—Eating disorders

—Eczema

—Edema of the feet

— Elbow pain

— Eyelids puffy

— Emphysema

—Enuresis (bed wetting)

—Erratic disruptive behavior

—Excessive appetite

__RATING   SYMPTOMS__

— Excessive drooling

— Excessive flatulence

— Excessive salivation

— Excessive sweating

— Exercise-induced asthma

— Failing memory

— Fainting spells

— Fatigue

— Fever of unknown origin

— Feels insecure

— Fibromyalgia

— Fibrocystic breast

— Food craving

— Food sensitivity

—Forgetfulness

— Formaldehyde allergy

— Frequent repetitive activity

— Frequent bronchitis

— Frequent ear infection

— Frequent flu's and colds.

— Frequent infections

— Frequent pneumonia

— Frequent sore throat

— Frequent sweating

— Frequent urination

RATING   SYMPTOMS

— Gags easily

— Gallstones

— Gastric distress

— Gastric ulcer

— General body aches

— General fatigue

— General itching

— Glaucoma

— Greasy food upsets

— Groin pain

— Growing pains

— Hay-fever

— Hair loss

— Hair pulling

— Halitosis

— Hand flicking

— Head banging

— Headache/afternoon

— Headache/migraine

— Headache over the eyes

— Headaches/sinus

— Headache/morning

— Headaches under the eyes

— Hearing loss

— Hearing decreased

RATING   SYMPTOMS

— Heartburn

— Heart irregularities

— Hemorrhoids

— Herpes Genital

— Herpes Zoster

— Hepatitis

— High altitude problem

— High blood pressure

— High cholesterol

— Hives

— Hoarseness

— Holds on to people and objects.

— Hot flashes

— Hungry between meals

— Hyperactivity

— Hypoglycemia

— Impaired ability to role-play

— Impaired speech

— Impaired peer relationships

— Impulsivity

— Increased sex drive

— Increased thirst

— Indigestion

— Infertility

— Internal tremor

RATING   SYMPTOMS

— Insomnia

— Irregular periods

— Irritability

— Irritable bowels

— Itchy eyes

— Jock itch

— Joint pains

— Keyed up, fails to calm down

— Knee pains

— Labored breathing

— Leaky gut syndrome

— Learning disabilities

— Light sensitivity

— Listlessness

— Loss of taste
— Loose stools

— Loud talk

— Low backache

— Low blood pressure

— Low body temperature

— Low libido

— Lump in the breast

— Lump in the throat

— Lupus

— Lymph node tenderness

— Metallic taste in the mouth

RATING   SYMPTOMS

— Mid backache

— Migrating pains

— Milk causes discomfort

— Mood swings

— Mucus in the throat

— Multiple sclerosis

— Muscle cramps at night

— Muscle pain

— Muscle spasms

— Nasal polyps

— Nausea

— Neck pains

— Nervous stomach

— Neuralgia

— Night sweats

— Nose-bleed

— Neuropathies

— Numbness anywhere in the body

— Obsessive behavior

— Ovarian cyst

— Pain between shoulders

— Pain on the heels

— Pain anywhere in the body without reason

— Panic attacks

— Paranoia

Say Good-bye to Headaches

RATING   SYMPTOMS

— Parasitic infestation

— Parrot-like talking

— Phobias

— Picking at skin.

— Pre menstrual pains or discomfort

— Poor appetite

— Poor concentration

— Poor memory

— Post nasal drip

— Premature graying

— Prone to infections

— Prostate troubles

— Psoriasis

— Recurrent prostatitis

— Red blood cells low

— Red blood cells high

— Red eyes

— Repeated dental infection

— Restless leg syndrome

— Reflex sympathetic dystrophy

— Ring worm

— Ringing in the ears

— Sadness

— Sand-like feeling in the eyes

— Sciatic neuralgia

RATING   SYMPTOMS

— scleroderma

— Seizures

— Sensitivities to any chemicals

— Sensitive to cold

— Sensitive to heat

— Sensitivities to weather change

— Shoulder pain

— Short term memory loss

— Shortness of breath

— Sighs frequently

— Sinusitis

— Skin problems

— Sleep apnea

— Sleepy during the day

— Slow pulse

— Slow starter

— Smell-decreased

— Sneezing attacks

— Sore throat

— Startles easily

— Strokes

— Strong lights irritates

— Swollen joints, ankles

— Thickening skin

— Thinning skin

RATING   SYMPTOMS

— Throat constriction

— Thyroid problem

— Tightness in the chest

— Tingling around the mouth

— Tingling anywhere in the body

— Tourette's syndrome

— Tires too easily

— Toxicity to heavy metal

— Toxicity to pesticides

— Ulcerative colitis

— Uncontrollable body movements

— Unable to fall asleep at night

— Unable to go back to sleep upon wakening

— Unable to sleep for long hours without waking

— Unexplained chest pain

— Unexplained pain in the body

— Unreasonable anger

— Unrefreshing sleep

— Unusual weight loss

— Upper backaches

— Urinary tract disorder

— Urination difficult

— Urine amount decreased

— Urine amount increased

— Uterine polyp

RATING   SYMPTOMS

— Vaginal discharge

— Varicose veins

— Vision problems

— Vomiting frequently

— Vulvodynia

— Vertigo

— Warts

— Weak nails

— Wake up during the night

— Watery eyes

— Weight gain for no reason

— Weight loss

— White blood cells low

— White blood cells high

— White spots

— Worrier

— Yeast infections

— Other

Say Good-bye to Headaches

CHAPTER 2

Categories of Allergies

A llergic reactions can be grouped according to the clinical manifestations of the person with allergies.

1.   People suffering from food allergies:

They have no seasonal symptoms, but suffer from varying numbers of unusual or unpleasant physical, physiological or emotional symptoms whenever they eat any food with some chemicals (for example, foods prepared with colorings, food additives, monosodium glutamate, etc.).

2.   People suffering from chemical allergies through external sources:

They have no unusual symptoms if they do not come in contact with any chemicals. They can be happy and healthy when they live in a natural environment surrounded by natural life, eating organically grown, unprocessed food. But, whenever they come near or in contact with any chemicals they are sensitive to, they suffer from a varying number of unusual or unpleasant physical, physiological, or emotional symptoms. As long as they wear or use 100% cotton, silk or any natural fabrics, they function well.

3. People suffering from chemical allergies from internal sources:

This group of people react to their own body secretions (sweat, urine, feces, mucous, semen, tears and saliva), body parts (hair and nails), different organs (stomach, spleen, lungs, kidney, liver, heart, brain, etc.). The body's defense mechanism is derailed, and the body makes antibodies against its own tissues and/ or fluids. The immune system attacks the body that it inhabits, which eventually causes damage or alteration to its own cells, tissues, organs and functions. Such damage results in cancer, abnormal tissue growths and tumors, kidney failure, organ failure, hearing loss, poor vision, heart attacks, liver failure, cataract, adrenal depletion, diabetes, thyroid malfunctions, etc.

4. People allergic to natural environmental allergens:

These people have frequent allergic symptoms such as tearing from the eyes, sneezing, wheezing, asthma, upper respiratory disturbances, fatigue, irritability, hay-fever symptoms during pollen season. They also show allergies to cotton, natural materials, but feel reasonably well for the rest of the year if they avoid natural products made from natural substances.

5. People suffering from allergies to animals and other humans:

These people have no allergies to food, drinks or the materials around them. They react to the electromagnetic energy of other living beings, which makes them allergic to other human beings, like their mother, father, spouse, brother, sister, children, partners, employee and employer. They can also have allergies to pets, cats, dogs, insects, bees, ants, etc.

6   People with emotional allergies:

The people in this group have allergies to the actions and interactions of everyday life. They may be allergic to their own: thoughts or feelings (fear, anger, self-esteem, creativity, power, self-worth, inferiority, superiority, etc.); concepts: ("I can never get healthy," "I can never lose weight," or "I can never make enough money," etc.); a memory of a certain incidence (such as nightmares, fear or anxiety while driving due to a memory of a highway auto accident that happened 10 years ago); emotions, like hating jobs or obsessions with careers (teaching, acting, cooking, gardening, writing, shopping, etc.), shop lifting, and interactions (fighting with co-workers, classmates, boss or teachers). Some allergic people enjoy going against rules and regulations, acting against the norm in situations or disobeying authorities (running red lights when the police is not watching, etc.)

7. People with combination allergies:

This group of people react to what seems to be an infinite number of combinations of food, pollens, chemicals, other humans, animals, thoughts, memories and concepts.

8. People who are universal reactors:

This group has multiple chemical sensitivities and suffer from severe reactions to all of the above allergens. They generally suffer from many other health problems. They are grouped as ecologically and environmentally ill. Ecological illness is the result of adverse reactions to substances in the air, water, food, living environment, work environments, and chemicals. These people do not feel safe anywhere.

It is rare to see people fall in any one group. Usually, people suffer symptoms from two or more groups.

CATEGORIES OF ALLERGENS

Common allergens are generally classified into nine basic categories based primarily on the method in which they are contacted, rather than the symptoms they produce.

1. Inhalants

2. Ingestants

3. Contactants

4. Injectants

5. Infectants

6. Physical agents

7. Genetic factors

8. Molds and fungi

9. Emotional Stressors

Allergens from Everyday Use that Can Trigger Headaches in Sensitive individuals

Acetic acid
Acrylic nails
After-shave lotion
Air conditioners
Air filters
Air freshener
Air pollution
Air purifiers
Alarm clock
Alcoholic beverages
Aluminum
Amalgam
Ammonia
Anti-bacterials
Antibiotics
Anti-depressants
Antiperspirants
Anything around the bed
Appearance enhancers
Aroma
Arsenic
Asbestos
Aspartame
Auto-detailing chemicals
Automobile exhaust
Bacteria
Bath accessories
Batteries
Bed
Bed linen
Bed pillow
Bed pillow cover
Bedroom materials
Bedstead

Benzene
Benzyl benzoate
Bleach
Blood
Body and hand lotion
Body creme
Body wash
Bodycare products
Books
Borax
Bottled drinking water (Check each time when you buy a new batch)
Braces & retainers
Brominated compounds
Boron
Building materials
Cadmium
Caffeine
Camphor
Candida
Cane products
Car deodorizer
Car smell
Carbon dioxide
Carbon monoxide
Carpet
Carpet chemicals
Carpet dust
Cars
Cat liter
Central heating
Ceramic tiles & products

Say Good-bye to Headaches

Charcoal
Chemicals from work or home
(kitchen, bathroom, and pool)
Cosmetics
Chloramines
Chlorine
Cigar smoke
Cleaning materials like mops
Cleansing supplies
Clorox
Cooking smells
Copying ink
Correction fluids
Cosmetics you or other family
members use
Crude oil: hard plastics, soft
plastics, synthetic fabrics,
formaldehyde, newspaper,
newspaper ink.
Cutting board
Dander
Dandruff
DDT
Deodorants
Deodorizers
Detergents
Diesel
Dioxin - (newspaper, paper
products, pesticides)
Dish washing soap, liquid
Down pillow
Drinking water
Drinks (any other)
Dry cleaning chemicals
Dry wall material
Dust
Dust mites
Dyes

EDTA
Electromagnetic radiation
Environmental substances (grass,
weeds, trees, pollens, flowers,
sand)
Equipment usage (Exercise
machines, C-pap machines, room
humidifier, etc.)
Ethylene gas
Fabric softener
Fabrics
Face cream
Fiberglass
Fillers in seats and cushions of
sofa and cars, pillows, stuffed
toys
Fire smoke
Flame retardents
Flavored drinks
Flea collars
Florescent light
Flour dust (used in baking and
cooking)
Fluoride
Food additives
Food chemicals
Food colorings
Food combining
Food flavorings
Foods from other source (TV
dinners, instant soups)
Foods with chemical sprays
Formaldehyde
Formic acid
Fragrances
Fresh food
Fruit Chemicals

Fumes
Fumigants
Fungi
GABA
Gasoline
Genetically modified foods
Geopathic stress
Gloss-finished brochures
Glossy paper
Glossy pictures and photos
Glues
Hair spray
Handwash
Head board
Heavy metals
Herbicides
Herbs and spices
Histamine
House dust
Housecleaning chemicals
Household cleaning products
House-plants
Ice cream
Illicit drugs
Immunization
In-car pollution
Indoor pollution
Industrial dust
Industrial waste
Insect bites and stings
Insecticides
Insulation
Irritants
Jams
Jelly and marmalades
Jewelry
Jewelry cleaning solution
Kava kava

Kelp
Laminates
Latex (elastics, stretch pants, socks, cosmetic applicators, gloves)
Lead
Lints
Lipstick
Liquid paper
Low level ozone
Magnets
Malic acid
Mannitol
Markers
Mattresses
Medications (prescription medication, over-the-counter medication, medicinal skin creams)
Methanol
Methylene chloride
Microorganisms (bacteria, viruses, parasites)
Microwaves
Milk and milk products
Mobile phone accessories
Mercury
Mobile phones
Mold
Mold spores
Monosodium glutamate [msg]
Moss
Moth repellants
Mothballs
Mouthwash
Naphthalene
Natural cosmetics
Natural dishwashing liquid

Say Good-bye to Headaches

Natural handwash
Natural paints
Natural products
Natural toothpowder
New car smell
Newspaper
Nickel
Nicotine
Noxious chemicals
Noxious fumes
Nuclear power
Office furniture
Office machines
Office products
Oils
Organic clothing
Organic foods
Organic paints
Organic products
Organophosphates
Ozone
Packaging material
Paint
Paint strippers
Paint thinner
Pajamas
Paper products
Paper products (newspaper, toilet paper, books, bills, paper money)
Paraffins
Parasympathetic nerves
PBB (polybrominated biphnenyl)
PBDE (Polybromodiphenyl ethers)
PCB (Polychlorinated biphenyls)
Personal clothing and products: Pant, Shirt, Undergarments, nylons, wool, night time clothing, sanitary napkins, leather belt, leather bag, shoes, slippers, toothpaste, mouth wash; cosmetics, after shave, makeup, lipstick, body lotion, perfume, antiperspirant, soap, detergent, smell.

Pesticides: malathion, ant-bait, insecticides, insect sprays, herbicides.

Perfume mix: all types of perfume
Pesticides
Pets
Phenylalanine
Phosphates
Photocopiers
Picture frame on the wall
Plastics (household products, house-wares, utility products, cosmetic applicators, phones, computer, key board, mouse, mouse pad, containers, electrical outlet covers, lids of vitamin containers, hard plastics, soft plastics, saran wrap, freezer bags, shopping bags, and various types of bags)
Plastic toys
Plastics-soft & hard
Polish
Pollen
Pollutants
Polysorbate
Polystyrene
Polyvinyl chloride
Potpouri
Preservatives
Pressed wood
Quartz

Quartz crystals
Radiation
Radiators
Radioactivity
Radon
Recycled paper goods
Recycling
Refrigerators
Room deodorizers
Saccharin
Salicylates
Salt
Saturated fats
Scents
Scrubbers (foam, metal, vinyl or plastic scrubbers in the kitchen)
Shampoo and hair conditioners
sorbitol
Selenium
Serotonin
Shelf-life enhancers
Synthetic materials (polyester, acrylic, acetate, nylon, cotton, rayon, silk, other petrochemical-based fabrics, rugs and carpet),
Silica
Silicates
Silver
Skin creams
Smell of cigarette
Smells from chemicals
Smells from various sources (from cooking, frying, seasoning, perfume, outside air, bodily secretion, or discharge, body odor, decayed material, stale food, flowers, perfume or any smell of

cosmetics from the bed partner, hospital wards, changed dressings from surgical wounds, water from gutters, backwaters, smell of waste products, smell of stool, other discharge)
Smog
Smoking (cigarette, tobacco, wood smoke, fireplace smoke, smog, sugar cane field smoke, any other kind of smoke primary or secondary in origin, and smell of the same)
Soap
Soft drinks
Solvents
Stabilisers
Static electricity
Static ions
Sugar
Sulfites
Sulphates
Supplements (vitamins, minerals, diet products, herbal and homeopathic remedies and other supplements)
Sweeteners
Swimming pool water
Sympathetic nerves
Synthetic detergents
Synthetic materials (polyester, acrylic, acetate, nylon, cotton, rayon, silk, other petrochemical-based fabrics, rugs and carpet), silica
Talcum powder
Tap water
Tartaric acid

Say Good-bye to Headaches

Tartrazine
Taste enhancers
Television monitor control
Tetevision sets
The smell of coffee brewing, and cooking smells
Tobacco
Tooth brush
Tooth paste
Toxic chemicals
Toxic fumes
Triglycerides
Trihalomethane
Turpentine
Tyramines
Ultra-violet radiation
Uranium

Utensils
Vaccines
Varnish
Vinyl
Volatile organic compounds
Wall pictures
Water chemicals
Water dechlorinating salts
Water pollutants
Weed-killer
White-out
Wood cabinet
Wood furniture
Wood smoke
Wood tables
Wood works and products
Wooden floor

INHALANTS

Inhalants are those allergens that are contacted through the nose, throat and bronchial tubes. Examples of inhalants are microscopic spores of certain grasses, flowers, pollens, powders, smoke, cosmetics, perfumes and chemical fumes such as paint, insecticides, fertilizers, flour from grains, cooking smells, etc.

It is difficult to say that there is a typical or predictable allergic reaction, or set of reactions, in response to a given allergen. If there is a predictable response, however, it is in this general category of inhalants that it comes closest to being found.

Most of us have suffered the discomfort that comes from accidentally breathing a toxic substance. For example, when we smell chlorine gas from a bottle of common household bleach, our reaction is immediate and violent as our eyes water, noses run, and bronchial tubes go into spasm, making breathing difficult. This experiment can be duplicated over and over if we want a proof that bleach is directly responsible for a given set of reactions. Of course, most of us learn very quickly that it is the bleach that caused our discomfort, and we decide to be more careful in the future. The cause and effect of this phenomena can be easily understood by everyone, because the discomfort is most obvious and everyone knows the bleach was the culprit for the sudden upper respiratory reactions because the smell receptors were involved here. How do we explain when someone gets a sudden headache as described above but the culprit was not so obvious like the bleach because it did not irritate usual sensory receptors?

A 46-year old female had to attend frequent business dinners along with her husband and their clients. After an hour into the dinner meetings, she would begin to get the warning signs of other approaching migrains. Half-way through the functions she would excuse herself, take her prescription medication and leave the party immediately so that she could reach home before her migraines got control of her. For this reason she drove in a separate automobile so that her husband could stay back and entertain the guests. When she got home she would straight away go to bed and usually she would be OK in the morning.

She was not nervous about parties; in fact she was a very social person. She liked company and entertaining them. No one could explain why she got her migraines each time she attended dinner parties.

When I evaluated her using NAET testing procedures, I discovered that she was highly allergic to the dry cleaning chemicals. The clothes she wore for the parties were all dry-cleaned. The sensitivity to the chemicals triggered her migraines. After she was desensitized for the dry cleaning chemicals, she stopped having migraines at the parties. Now she can enjoy the parties from beginning to end without having to worry about leaving half-way through the functions.

Another female patient in her fifties suffered from severe migraines once a week, usually on Friday nights. By midnight of Friday she had to be driven to the emergency room for her usual injection. After she receives her usual injection she would return home to sleep it off in a noise-free, light-free room for the next two days. She would be OK for the rest of the week. Her once a week migraines continued for several years. Then she heard from her friend that there is a ray of hope for headache-free days through NAET. She immediately made an appointment and came to see me for an evaluation and possible treatment. Upon NAET evaluation, I found her headaches to be triggered by the smell of the hair chemicals she encountered on Friday afternoons at the hair salon. For many years she had gone for her hair appointments on Friday afternoons since that was the most convenient time for her since she did not work on Fridays. When she received the medication in the emergency room, her overactive nerves would calm down and she would sleep for several hours. By the time she wakes up, the annoying smell is forgotton by the nerves and she gets free from her head pains. As clockwork, her headache appeared at the same time every week on Friday nights. This created extreme fear in her not knowing the trigger for her once a week headache. She was afraid to leave town or to take a vacation. She was afraid to leave her home on Friday thinking that if she got the headache she wouldn't know which hospital to go for help. She did not want to get stranded at another city or town with her debilitating migraines.

She was treated for five basics and then for the hair chemicals (sample collected from the hair salon by the patient). She was desensitized for the hair chemicals three different times on three consecutive days. Then she was desensitized for the smell of the chemicals. She completed her treatments for the chemicals on Thursday. She went for her hair appointment on Friday as usual. The whole evening she kept waiting for her headache to appear. For the first time in years she went to bed on that Friday without a headache. She didn't have to visit emergency room again seeking treatment for headaches.

Jane carpooled with her friend to work from Monday through Friday. She complained of tension headache for half an hour to one hour each time she exited the car. Her physician referred her to me for possible desensitization of car chemicals (gasoline, etc.), because these chemicals were blamed until she came to me for an evaluation and possible treatment. On NAET evaluation, it was detected that her headaches were not due to car chemicals but the faint smell from the dry cleaning chemicals from her friend's clothes. After she was treated for the dry cleaning chemicals, she did not have tension headaches anymore.

This clearly points out that there is no typical response to allergens in the real world. If we are depending on allergies to produce a given set of responses for all people, we may misdiagnose and provide wrong treatments. We must remember that since we cannot duplicate and package a cause-and-effect responsive medication as antidote to handle all cases of poisoning from inhaling fern tree spores, or any other allergen, we must not oversimplify our treatment of patients who do not exhibit typical allergic symptoms, whatever we perceive them to be. Otherwise, we risk missing myriad potential reactions that may be produced in some people in response to their contacts with substances that are, for them, allergens.

ALLERGIC RHINITIS AND HEADACHES

Allergic rhinitis occurs in the late summer due to an individual's reaction to ragweeds and sage weeds or fresh flowers and grasses. Allergic rhinitis affects an estimated 40-50 million people in the United States. It produces severe headaches along with hay-fever like symptoms in environmentally sensitive people when they are exposed to pollens from trees, grasses, weeds or to airborne mold spores. It can be also caused by other substances like house dust, occupational dust (such as flour in the bakery, industrial dust, etc.), dust mites, animal dander, mold spores, contact with certain furniture, chalk powder, newspaper ink, paint, plastics, chemical sprays, soaps, perfumes, plastics, latex, and other chemical agents. Many patients with pollen allergies will also be allergic to certain foods, as well as to other inhalants and contactants. Allergic rhinitis is characterized by symptoms of headaches, watery discharge from the nose, eyes, and throat, loss of taste and smell, and other symptoms similar to those accompanying colds. The most common items found to cause allergic rhinitis are: sugar, carob, corn, wheat, beans, pineapple, tomato, banana and perfume. Often, these individuals also suffer from nasal polyps, which are swellings or growths of the mucus membrane that occur within the nostrils.

It is extremely important that these indivisuals consult an appropriate allergist knowledgeable in NAET when their symptoms begin. Allergic rhinitis has a tendency to become increasingly severe with each season. Untreated patients are also likely to accumulate new allergens, as well as encountering increased sensitivity in their reactions.

Prompt NAET desensitization treatment of these allergies greatly decreases the likelihood of getting headaches from allergic rhinitis.

SINUSITIS AND HEADACHES

Sinusitis is inflammation or infection of any of the four groups of sinus cavities in the skull, which open into the nasal passages. Sinusitis is not the same as rhinitis, although the two may be associated and their symptoms may be similar. The terms "sinus trouble" or "sinus congestion" are sometimes wrongly used to mean congestion of the nasal passages. Most cases of nasal congestion are not associated with sinusitis. If sinusitis is allowed to continue, it can eventually turn into asthma. Most sinusitis patients suffer from severe headaches.

A 34-year-old housewife who loved to cook would end up in the Emergency room for treatment of migraines every time she cooked Italian food. She never ate the food for fear of getting headaches. She only cooked for the family. After she gets treated in the emergency room, she usually felt better within four hours. Nobody suspected an allergy to the smell from cooking as a reason for her migraines. She was seen in our office. Upon NAET evaluation, it was discovered that the smell of the garlic in cooking triggered here migraines. After he was successfully treated for Garlic, not only can she smell the garlic now, but she can also cook italian food with lots of garlic and eat with the family without having any trace of headaches.

I have treated many men and women who began having migraines after they got married. The culprits were traced to the partner's clothes, perfume, hair sprays, after-shave, body odor, etc. In some cases I have found the allergy between the husband and wife causing one or both of them to suffer from migraine-like headaches. Usually the successful completion of NAET treatments prevent further migraines.

INGESTANTS

Ingestants are allergens that are contacted in the normal course of eating a meal or that enter the system in other ways through the mouth and find their way into the gastrointestinal tract. These include: foods, drinks, condiments, drugs, beverages, chewing gums, vitamin supplements, etc. All these are potential allergens that trigger headaches at any time in sensitive individuals.

Sulfites are preservatives used by the fast food industry. The intention was to maintain freshness (or at least the appearance of freshness and flavor) as these vegetables sit out in display cases for long periods of time. Unfortunately, sulfites are salt derivatives of sulfuric acid, which many chemically sensitive persons are highly allergic to and produce headaches.

Literally any substance we eat can become an allergen for someone who is sensitive to any ingredient in the product and trigger a headache. New substances are being introduced into our diets that preserve color, flavor and extend the shelf life of our foods. Some additives used in foods as preservatives have caused severe health problems. Some artificial sweeteners cause mysterious problems in some sensitive people and may cause various types of headaches. Most of these additives are harmless to most people but can produce headaches in people with sensitivity to the item.

Some people get their headaches when they are late to eat. When their blood glucose lowers for some reason, they begin to have headaches. These people should correct their problem at an early age, otherwise they are good candidates to develop diabetes or similar conditions in the future. Headache is only a warning sign for such people.

Allergy to corn is one of today's most common allergies, especially in people with headaches. Unfortunately, corn starch is found in almost every processed food and some toiletries and drugs too. Chinese food, baking soda, baking powder, and toothpaste contain large amounts of cornstarch. It is the binding product in almost all vitamins and pills, including aspirin and Tylenol. Corn syrup is the natural sweetener in many of the products we ingest, including soft drinks. Corn silk is found in cosmetics and corn oil is used as a vegetable oil. For sensitive people this food adds another nightmare.

Other common ingredients in many preparations that people may react severely to are the various gums (acacia gum, xanthine gum, karaya gum, etc.). Numerous gums are used in candy bars, yogurt, cream cheese, soft drinks, soy sauce, barbecue sauce, fast food products, macaroni and cheese, etc.

Tyramine is a common trigger for migraine and other headaches. Some people with migraine have a genetic deficiency of the enzyme, which metabolises tyramine, and an excessive intake will trigger an attack. Tyramine is naturally seen in these following foods: banana, bass, bean(soya), beef, beer, cheese (more in aged cheese), cottage cheese, chicken, cocoa, chocolate, egg, oyster, pea, plum, pork, potato, sweet potato, prune, raisin, spinach, tomato, walnut, and yeast. According to NAET theory, an allergy of one's body towards a particular enzyme (in this case, the enzyme to digest tyramine) prevents the body from producing that particular enzyme within the body leading to a genetic deficiency as we see in many cases. After a successful NAET desensitization for tyramine, body will begin to produce the required enzyme for the digestion of tyramine as and when necessary on its own (without any supplementation) and thus the future consumption of tyramine will not trigger migraines. Taking enzyme supplements without clearing the allergy may help to mask the symptoms temporarily but it does not solve the underlying problem of the body's inability to produce the enzyme as and when needed.

Food coloring triggers headaches among sensitive people. Young school-going children consume various food colorings in large quantity in various forms: ice cream, candies, chewing gums, dry cereals, etc. Many children suffer from headaches, hyperactivity, poor concentration, irritability, etc. after they consume attractive cereals filled with various food dyes.

Carob, a staple in many health food products, is another item that causes brain irritability and headaches among allergic people. Many health-conscious people are turning to natural food products in which carob is used as a chocolate and cocoa substitute. It is also used as a natural coloring or stiffening agent in soft drinks, cheeses, sauces, etc. We discovered that some of the causes of "holiday flu" and suicide attempts are allergies to carob, chocolate, and turkey.

If you have allergies you must look for these following ingredients and additives in the food products you buy from the market. These have triggered headaches in many people. If you are allergic to these items, find a NAET practitioner and get yourself desensitized through NAET treatments. Or else avoid them to prevent headaches.

Please read the labels. Manufacturers usually list these items on the cover of the product-container.

Acetic Acid (sodium acetate and sodium diacetate). This is a common food additive. This is the acid of vinegar. Acetic acid is used as an acidic flavoring agent for pickles, sauces, catsups, mayonnaise, wine, foods that are preserved in vinegar, some soft drinks, processed cheese, baked goods, cheese spreads, sweet and sour drinks and soups. It is also naturally found in apples, cocoa, coffee, wine, cheese, grapes, and other over-ripened fruits. If your child gets allergic reaction to these natural foods he/she may be allergic to acetic acid.

Agar (Seaweed extract): This is a polysaccharide that comes from several varieties of algae and it can turn like a gel if you dissolve it in water. So this is used in ice cream, jellies, preserves, icings, laxatives, used as a thickening agent in milk, cream, and used as gelatin (vegetable form). This is a safe additive, but if your child is allergic to sea foods you may need to eliminate the allergy for this.

Albumin (cow milk-albumin): Many children are allergic to albumin in the milk. Researchers have found children/people who are allergic to milk albumin are at high risk to get any of these disorders: ADD, ADHD, Autism, bipolar diseases, schizophrenia, and other allergy-related brain disorders. NAET can desensitize you for milk-albumin.

Aldicarb: It is an organic chemical water pollutant, seen often in city water. When the concentration of this chemical gets high in the city water, many people get sick with gastrointestinal disorders, like nausea, vomiting, pain, bloating, stomach flu, etc. Boiling the water for 30 minutes could help reduce the reaction. If your child is not allergic to apple cider vinegar, adding two-three drops of vinegar in eight ounces of water might help.

Alginates (Alginic acid, algin gum, ammonium, calcium, potassium, and sodium alginates, propylene glycol alginates): Most of these are natural extracts of seaweed and used in the food industry primarily as stabilizing agents.

Propylene glycol is an antifreeze. This is supposed to be a safe solvent, used in food preparation, especially in ice creams. Alginates help to retain water. It helps to prevent ice crystal formation; helps uniform distribution of flavors through foods. They add smoothness and texture to the products and are used in ice creams, custards, chocolates, chocolate milk, cheese, salad dressings, jellies, confections, cakes, icings, jams, and some beverages.

Aluminum Salts (alum hydroxide, alum potassium sulfate, sodium alum phosphate, alum ammonium sulfate, and alum calcium silicate).: Aluminum salts are used as a buffer in various products. This helps to balance the acidity. Used as an astringent to keep canned produce firm, to lighten food texture, and used as an anti-caking agent.

Sodium aluminum phosphate is used in baking powder and in self-rising flours. Alum is used as a clarifier for sugar and as a hardening agent. Aluminum hydroxide is used as a leavening agent in baked goods. It is a strong alkali agent that can be toxic but when used in small amounts it is fairly safe. It is also used in antiperspirants and antacids. Aluminum ammonium sulfate is used as an astringent, and neutralizing agent in baking powder and cereals. It can cause burning sensation to the mucous membranes. Overuse of aluminum products may lead to aluminum toxicity and it can affect the brain chemistry. Other sources of aluminum are cookware, deodorants, antacids, aluminum foils, cans and containers.

Benzoates (sodium benzoate): Benzoic acid occurs naturally in anise, berries, black olive, blueberries, broccoli, cauliflower, cherry bark, cinnamon, cloves, cranberries, ginger, green grapes, green peas, licorice, plums, prunes, spinach, and tea. Benzoic acid or sodium benzoate is commonly used as a preservative in food processing. This is used as a flavoring agent in chocolate, orange, lemon, nut, and other flavors in beverages, baked products, candies, ice creams, and chewing gums and also used as a preservative in soft drinks, margarine, jellies, juices, pickles, and condiments. This is also used in perfumes and cosmetics to prevent spoilage by microorganisms. Benzoic acid is a mild antifungal agent. It is metabolized by the liver. Large amount of benzoic acid or benzoates can cause intestinal disturbances, can irritate the eyes, skin, and mucous membranes. This causes eczema, acne and other skin conditions in sensitive people.

Cal. Proprionate: (sodium proprionate and proprionic acid): These are found in dairy products, cheese, breads, cakes, baked goods and chocolate products, They are used as preservatives and mold inhibitors. They reduce the growth of molds and some bacteria. This is often seen as an additive in these products: Baked products, breads, rolls, cakes, cup cakes, processed cheese, chocolate products, preserves, jellies, and butter.

Cal. Silicate: Used as an anticaking agent in products, table salt and other foods preserved in powder form used as a moisture control agent.

Carbamates: These pesticides are used widely in many places. Their toxicity is slightly lesser than some other pesticides like organochlorines. They are known to produce birth defects.

Source: pesticide-sprayed foods.

Carbon Monoxide: CO is an odorless, colorless gas that competes with oxygen for hemoglobin. The affinity of CO for hemoglobin is more than 200-fold greater than that of oxygen. CO causes tissue hypoxia. Headache is one of the first symptoms, followed by confusion, decreased visual acuity, tachycardia, syncope, metabolic acidosis, retinal hemorrhage, coma, convulsions, and death.

Carbon monoxide can be encountered via these following sources: Driving through heavy traffic, damaged gas range, leaky valves of the gas line, exhaust pipes, living in a closed up room for long time, trapped firewood smoke, smoke inhalation from being in a closed, running car, an automobile kept running in closed garage for hours, exhaust from autos and other machinery, etc.

Casein: Milk protein. Also used in prepared foods, candies, protein shakes, etc.

EDTA: This is a very efficient polydentate chelator of many divalent or trivalent cations including calcium. This is used primarily in lead poisoning. This is toxic to the kidneys. Adequate hydration is necessary when you take this in any form.

Ethylene gas (used on fruits, especially on green bananas).

Food Bleach: Most of these are used in bleaching flour products. Benzoil peroxides, chlorine dioxides, nitrosyl chlorides, potassium bromate, mineral salts, potassium iodate, ammonium sulfate, ammonium phosphate, are the most commonly used food bleaches. They whiten the flour. They also improve the appearance. Whatever they are using should be listed on the labels. Sometimes more than one item is used for better benefit.

Formic Acid: This is a caustic, colorless, forming liquid. Naturally seen in ants (ant bite), synthetically produced and used in tanning and dyeing solutions, fumigants and insecticides. This is also used as an artificial flavoring in food preparations.

Malic Acid: A colorless, highly water soluble, crystalline substance, having a pleasant sour taste, and found in apples, grapes, rhubarb, and cactus. This substance is found to be very effective in reducing general body aches. If you are allergic to it, then you can get severe body ache.

Mannan: Polysaccharides of mannose, found in various legumes and in nuts. Allergy to this factor in dried beans causes fibromyalgia-like symptoms in sensitive people.

Mannitol: It is hexahydric alcohol, used in renal function testing to measure glomerular filtration. Used intravenously as an osmotic diuretic.

Salicylic Acid: Amyl, phenyl, benzyl, and methyl salicylates).

A number of foods including almonds, apples, apricots, berries, plums, cloves, cucumbers, prunes, raisins, tomatoes, and wintergreen. Salicylic acid made synthetically by heating phenol with carbon dioxide is the basis of acetyl salicylic acid. Salicylates are also used in a variety of flavorings such as strawberry, root beer, spice, sarsaparilla, walnut, grapes, and mint.

Succinic Acid: Found in meats, cheese, fungi, and many vegetables with its distinct tart, acid taste. This is also found in asparagus, broccoli, beets, and rhubarb.

Talc (magnesium silicate): Talc is a silica chalk that is used in coating, polishing rice and as an anticaking agent. It is used externally on the body surface to dry the area. Talc is thought to be carcinogenic. It may contain asbestos particles. White rice is polished and coated with it.

Tartaric Acid: This is a flavor enhancer. It is a stabilizer.

Commonly seen Water Chemicals (in drinking water). are as follows: Alum sulfate, ammonium chloride, benzene, carbon tetrachloride, chlorine, DDT, ferric chloride, gasoline, heavy metals (mercury, silver, zinc, arsenic, lead, copper), organochlorides, organophosphates, PCBs, pesticides, petroleum products, Sodium hydroxide, toluene, and xylene.

Commonly seen Water pollutants: There are many water pollutants we see in our water. Some of them get filtered out by the time we receive it in our tap. Most of these pollutants still remain in small amounts. Some of these are inorganic water pollutants like: arsenic, asbestos, cadmium, chromium, copper, cyanide, Lead, mercury, nickels, nitrates, nitrosamines, selenium, silica, silver, and zinc.

Organic chemical water pollutants: 1,2, dichloroethane, 2,4,5,T, 2,4,-D., aldicarb, benzene, carbon tetrachloride, chloroform, DDT, dibromo-chloropropane (DBCP), dichlorobenzene, dioxane, endrin, ethylene dibromide (EDB), gasoline, lindane, methoxychlor, polychlorinated biphenyls (PCB), polynuclear aromatic hydrocarbon (PAH), tetrachloroethylene, toluene, toxaphene, trichloromethane, trichloroethylene (TCE), vinyl chloride, MTBE (Methyl tertiary butyl ether is a gasoline additive), and xylene.

Some people with extreme sensitivity to these pollutants suffer from repeated migraines and other types of headaches with exposure to the above chemicals.

CONTACTANTS

Contactants produce their effect by direct contact with the skin. They include the well-known poison oak, poison ivy, poison sumac, cats, dogs, rabbits, cosmetics, soaps, skin cremes, detergents, rubbing alcohol, gloves, hair dyes, various types of plant oils, chemicals such as gasoline, dyes, acrylic nails, nail polish, fabrics, formaldehyde, furniture, cabinets, etc. Any contact with any of these items can trigger headaches in sensitive people.

Allergic reactions to contactants can be different in each person, and may include migraine headaches and other types of headaches.

Woolen clothes may also cause allergic headaches. We have seen people who cannot wear wool without breaking out in rashes. Some people who are sensitive to wool also react to creams with lanolin base, since lanolin is derived from sheep wool. Some people can be allergic to cotton socks, orlon socks, or woolen socks with symptoms of knee pain, etc. People can also be allergic to carpets and drapes that could cause knee pains and joint pains.

We had a few other female patients who were allergic to their panty hose and suffered from headaches, leg cramps, high blood pressure, swollen legs, psoriasis, and persistent yeast infections. Toilet paper and paper towels also cause problems, mimicking yeast infections in many people. Many women are allergic to their synthetic bras and to feminine tampons. There are reports from women-sufferers that probably their allergy to antiperspirant or usage of synthetic bras caused some of them to have various types of headaches.

Many people are allergic to underarm deodorants and antiperspirants, causing headaches, skin rashes, irritation of the skin, dermatitis, boils, infections, lymph gland swelling and pain. The chemicals in the antiperspirants and deodorants are toxic and carcinogenic to some people. These products do their intended job, that is to prevent sweating, by blocking the sweat glands. That could lead to inflammation of the sweat glands, and constant irritation and inflammation can lead to more chronic disorders like breast cancer.

Many people are allergic to crude oils and their derivatives, which include plastic and synthetic rubber products. Can you imagine the difficulty of living in this modern society, trying to be completely free from products made of crude oil? A person would literally be immobilized. The phones we use, the naugahyde chairs we sit on, the milk containers we use, the polyester fabrics we wear, most of the face and body creams we use, all are made from a common product - crude oil! Many people suffer from headaches when they associate with any of the above.

Food items, normally classified as ingestants, may also act as contactants on persons who handle them constantly over time. Cooks who knead the wheat flour daily could suffer from migraines and other types of headaches because they were allergic to the grains and the flour they use in cooking. People who cut vegetables and pack them in the grocery stores could suffer from various types of headaches from the allergy to the vitamin C from the vegetables. Some people suffer from fibromyalgia and chronic fatigue by continuous exposure to certain vegetables and food products like cutting and canning peppers or onions.

Other career-produced headaches have been diagnosed for cooks, waiters, grocery-store keepers, clerks, gardeners, etc. Virtually no trade or skill is exempt from contracting allergens.

INJECTANTS

Allergens are injected into the skin, muscles, joints and blood vessels in the form of various serums, antitoxins, vaccines and drugs. As in any other allergic reaction, the injection of a sensitive drug into the system runs the risk of producing dangerous allergic reactions. To the sensitive person, the drug actively becomes a poison, with the same effect as an injection of arsenic and cause headaches.

Most of us do not often consider an insect bite in the same way as we would an injection received from a physician or a member of the staff, but the result is quite the same. At the point of the bite, a minute amount of the body fluid (saliva) of the insect is injected into the body. These fluids may be incidental to the bite, but very capable of causing severe headaches in some people.

INFECTANTS

Infectants are allergens that produce their effect by causing a sensitivity to an infectious agent, such as bacteria. For example, when tuberculin bacteria is introduced as part of a diagnostic test to determine a patient's sensitivity and/or reaction to that particular agent, an allergic reaction may result. This may occur during skin patch, or scratch tests done in the normal course of allergy testing in traditional Western medical circles.

Infectants differ from injectants as allergens because of the nature of the allergenic substances; that is, the substance is a known injectant and is limited in the amount administered to the patient. A slight prick of the skin introduces the toxin through the epidermis and a pox or similar harmless skin lesion will erupt if the patient is allergic or reactive to that substance. For most people, the pox soon dries up and forms a scab which eventually drops off, without much discomfort. However, for those individuals who are reactive to these tests, it is not uncommon to experience fainting, nausea, fever, swelling (not only at the scratch site but over the whole body), respiratory distress, headaches, etc.

In other words, the introduction of an allergen into the chemically sensitive person's system runs the potential risk of causing a severe reaction, regardless of the reason or the amount of the toxic substance used. Great care must be taken in the administration of tests that are designed to produce an allergic reaction.

Various vaccinations and immunizations may also produce severe allergic reactions in sensitive people. Some children after they receive their usual immunization get very sick physically and emotionally. Many children suffering from repeated headaches also suffer from attention deficit and hyperactive disorders, learning disability and behavioral problems. After successful desensitization with NAET, they have returned to normalcy (The journal of NAET Energetics and Complementary Medicine, (2)(2), 2006).

It should be noted that bacteria, virus, etc. are contacted in numerous ways. Our casual contact with objects and people exposes us daily to dangerous contaminants and possible illnesses. When our autoimmune systems are functioning properly, we pass off the illness without notice. When our systems are not working at maximum performance levels, we experience infections, fevers, etc.

From a strictly allergenic standpoint, however, contact with an injectant does not produce the expected reaction all the time, rather a more typical allergic reaction may take place. Some patients get signs and symptoms of 'flu' each year soon after they receive the 'flu' shots. One of my patients used to get different types of headaches and other symptoms each year after receiving the said vaccination for the influenza. We decided to desensitize her for the injectant a week prior to actually receiving the vaccinations. Her headaches arising as the after-effect of flu vaccinations have stopped completely. For the past six years she was not bothered by headaches after the usual flu shots.

PHYSICAL AGENTS

Heat, cold, sunlight, dampness, drafts or mechanical irritants may also cause allergic reactions and are known as physical allergens. When the patient suffers from more than one allergy, physical agents can affect the patient greatly. If the patient has already consumed some allergic food item, then walks in cold air or drafts, she might develop upper respiratory problems, sore throat, asthma or joint pains, etc., depending on his/her tendency toward health problems. Some people are very sensitive to cold or heat, whether they have eaten any allergic food or not. Such cases are common.

John suffered from frequent migraines in the winter. When the summer comes he never had head pains. He was allergic to cold, iron and calcium.

Barbara, 42 year old nerse had experienced severe head-aches since she was a teanager. She was on hormone supple-ments, but nothing gave her relief. She was found to be allergic to her own hormones, salt, minerals and heat. After she was cleared for the allergy to the above items, her headaches dimin-ished greatly.

Jenny, 58, suffered from Raynaud's disease. The tip of her fingers remained dark blue on a cold day. She was allergic to cold, citrus fruits, and meat products. She felt better when she was cleared for the above items.

Many arthritic patients, asthma patients, migraine patients, PMS patients, and mental patients have exaggerated symptoms of headaches and other pains on cold, cloudy or rainy days. These types of patients could suffer from severe allergy to electrolytes, cold, or a combination of both.

Some patients react to heat or cold violently, getting aches and pains during a cloudy day, and icy cold hands and feet even if they are clad in multiple warm socks. These patients have hypo-functioning immune systems. When they finish the treatment pro-gram, they do not continue to feel cold or get sick with the heat or cold.

GENETIC CAUSES

Discovery of possible tendencies toward allergies carried over from parents and grandparents opens a large door to achieving optimum health. Most people inherit the allergic tendency from their parents or grandparents. Allergies can also skip generations and be manifested very differently in children.

Many people with various allergic manifestations respond well to the treatment of various disease agents that have been transmitted from parents.

Parents with rheumatic fever may transmit the disease to their offspring, but in the children the rheumatic fever agent may not be manifested in its original form. As example, Sara, 42, had severe migraines all her life. Her mother had rheumatic fever as a child. Treatment for rheumatic fever lessened her migraines.

A woman who suffered from bronchial asthma was cleared of her asthma when she was treated for pneumococcus, the bacterium responsible for pneumonia. Both of her parents had died of pneumonia soon after her birth.

Ray, a man of 44, responded well to the treatment for diphtheria, thus clearing his chronic bronchitis. He had inherited the tendency toward allergies from his mother, who almost died from diphtheria when she was seven. The reaction to diphtheria was manifested in him as bronchitis, sinusitis and arthritis.

MOLDS AND FUNGI

Molds and fungi are in a category by themselves, because of the numerous ways they are contacted as allergens in everyday life. They can be ingested, inhaled, touched or even, as in the case of Penicillin, injected. They come in the form of airborne spores, making up a large part of the dust we breathe or pick up in our vacuum cleaners; fluids such as our drinking water; as dark fungal growth in the corners of damp rooms; as athlete's foot; and in particularly obnoxious vaginal conditions commonly called "yeast infections." They grow on trees and in the damp soil. They are a source of food, as in truffles and mushrooms; of diseases such as ring worm and the aforementioned yeast infections, and of healing, as in the tremendous benefits mankind has derived from the drug Penicillin.

Reactions to these substances are as varied as other kinds of allergies. This is because they are a part of one of the largest known classifications of biological entities. Because of the number of ways they can be introduced into the human anatomy, the number of reactions are multiplied considerably. Fungi are parasites that grow on living as well as decaying organic matter. That means that some forms are found growing in the human anatomy. The problem of athlete's foot is a prime example.

Athlete's foot is a human parasite fungus that grows anywhere in the body, where the area is fairly moist and not exposed to sunlight or air. It is particularly difficult to eliminate, and treatment generally consists of a topical preparation, multiple daily cleansing of the area, a medicinal powder, and wearing light cotton socks to avoid further infection from dyes used in colored wearing apparel.

It is contracted by contact with the fungus and is often passed from person to person anywhere there is the potential for contact (i.e. gymnasiums, showers, locker rooms and other areas where people share facilities and walk barefoot), thus the name athlete's foot. If it is a real athlete's foot, it will clear with the NAET treatment. Certain allergies, like allergies to socks made of cotton, orlon, or nylon, etc., can mimic athlete's foot. In such cases, athlete's foot may not clear by using medications.

Allergies to cotton, orlon, nylon, or paper could result in the explosions of infections including Ascomycetes fungi (yeast) that women are finding so troublesome. Feminine tampons, toilet papers, douches, and deodorants can also cause yeast infections.

EMOTIONAL STRESSORS

Many times, the origin of physical symptoms can be traced back to some unresolved emotional trauma. Each cell in the body (meridians) has the capability to respond physically, physiologically and psychologically to our daily activities. When the vital energy flows evenly and uninterrupted through the energy pathways (acupuncture meridians), the body functions normally. When there is a disruption in the energy flow through the meridians (an increase or decrease), energy blockages can occur, causing various emotional symptoms in those particular meridians. According to Oriental medical theory, there are seven major emotions which can cause pathological health problems in people: sadness affects lung meridian, joy affects the heart, disgust affects the stomach, anger affects the liver, worry affects the spleen, fear affects the kidney, and depression affects the pericardium meridian. Please read chapter 5 for more information.

A 32-year-old female suffered from severe headaches whenever she did any cooking. Then she would be sick for the next three or four days. She was evaluated in our office and found that she suffered from a severe emotional trauma when she was four years old. She was a very hyperactive child. Her aunt who was a teenager was baby sitting. One day she put her in the chicken coup and locked her for over an hour. The aunt also threatened the child to spank her with the kitchen spatula if she cried or made any sound. The girl sat in the corner of the empty cage smelling the chicken waste for the fear of the beating with the large spatula. When her mother returned she found the child sitting in the empty chicken cage and silent tears flowing down the cheeks. Her aunt reported that it was impossible to control her due to her extreme hyperactivity and that was the only way she could keep her quite until her mother got home. Each time she went into the kitchen she spotted the spoons and spatula hanging in the wall. Her subconscious mind remembered the above childhood traumatic memory and her brain responded by giving her an instant excrutiating headache. Unable to do any cooking without triggering such headaches, she finally would give up and find salvation to her growling stomach in some restaurants.

After she was desensitized to this past trauma, she is able to cook food in her kitchen and able to eat home-cooked meals now. She also reported happily that she saved a lot of money by avoiding restaurants in the past year and with that saved money she was able to take a fourteen-day mediterranian cruise this year.

CHAPTER 3

Detecting Allergies

Allergic conditions occur much more frequently than most people realize. Every year there are more and more recognized cases of allergies in the United States. Statistics show that at least 50 percent of the population suffers from some form of allergy. Many people are interested in understanding the differences and/or the similarities of the methods of diagnosis, the effectiveness and length of treatment between traditional Western medicine and Oriental medicine. Since the purpose of this book is to provide information about the new treatment method of NAET®, more attention will be given to Oriental medicine.

With NAET®, it is extremely important for the patient to cooperate with the physician in order to obtain the best results. It is my hope that this chapter will help bring about a clearer understanding between allergists and their patients because, in order to obtain the most satisfactory results, both parties must work together as a team.

The first step in diagnosing a headache is to take a thorough patient history, including chief complaint, present history, past medical history, family history, social history, history of activities, hobbies and nutrition. It will be beneficial to obtain a thorough record of any past sensitivity reactions in the patient's family, tracing back two or three generations if possible. Various allergies can trigger headaches in sensitive individuals. The patient will be asked whether either parent suffers from headaches, ever suffered from any type of allergy. The practitioner will ask whether the patient's parents were unable to eat certain foods or professed to "hate" certain foods because of how the particular food made them feel; or had any allergic reactions such as hives, eczema, dermatitis, indigestion, constipation, nervous stomach, fat intolerance, lactose intolerance, sinusitis, runny nose, frequent colds or flu, mental illness, heart disorders, or any other conditions where an allergy may have been a contributing factor, whether or not recognized as such at the time.

The same questions are asked about the patient's other relatives: grandparents, aunts, uncles, brothers, sisters and cousins. An allergic tendency is not always inherited directly from the parents. It may skip generations, and manifest in nieces or nephews rather than in direct descendants.

The careful practitioner will also determine whether such diseases as tuberculosis, cancer, diabetes, rheumatic or glandular disorders exist or have ever occurred in the patient's family history. All of these facts help give the allergist a more complete picture of the hereditary characteristics of the patient. *Allergic tendency* is inherited. It may be manifested differently in different people. Unlike the tendency, an actual allergic condition, such as headaches is not always inherited. Parents may have had cancer or rheumatism, but the child can manifest that allergic inheritance as migraine headaches.

When the family history is complete, the allergist will need to look into the history of the patient's recent history of headaches. Some typical preliminary questions include: When did your first episode occur? Did your headache first occur when you were a child, or did you first notice the symptoms after you were fully grown? Did it occur after going through a certain procedure? For example, did it occur for the first time after a hair perm? One of my patients reported that her first migraine occurred for the first time half hour after she got her hair colored. She was allergic to the hair dye used in the coloring.

Once a careful history is taken, the allergist often discovers that the patient's first symptoms occurred following a certain exposure to an allergen. Next, the doctor will want to know the circumstances surrounding and immediately preceding the first symptoms. Typical questions will include: Did you change your diet or go on a special diet? Did you eat something that you hadn't eaten perhaps for two or three months? Do you eat one type of food repeatedly, every day? Did the symptoms follow a childhood illness (whooping cough, measles, chicken pox, diphtheria) or any immunization for such an illness? Did they follow some other illness, such as influenza, pneumonia, viral infection, or a major operation? Did the symptoms first appear at adolescence or after you had a baby? Were they first noticed after you acquired a cat, a dog, or even a bird? Did they appear after an automobile accident or any major physical or mental trauma? Did they appear after a lengthy exposure to the sun, a day at the beach or 18 holes of golf? Did they appear after receiving a gift for your birthday? Or after starting to use a new pair of socks, pants, shirt, after-shave, wrist watch, leather belt, leather shoes, a chair, furniture, certain shampoo, cosmetics? Did your symptoms begin after a new arrival in the house (a baby, a guest, a pet, etc.)?

Any one of these factors can be responsible for triggering a headache of any intensity. Therefore, it is very important to obtain full and accurate answers when taking a patient's medical history.

Other important questions also should relate to the frequency and occurrence of the sensitivity reaction-episodes. Although foods may be a factor, if the symptoms occur only at specific times of the year, the trouble is most likely due to pollens. Often a patient is sensitive to certain foods but has a natural tolerance that prevents sickness until the pollen sensitivity adds sufficient allergens to throw the body into an imbalance. If symptoms occur only on specific days of the week, they are probably due to something contacted or eaten on that particular day.

The causes of allergic attacks in different patients can, at first, appear to be random. Regular weekly attacks of migraines were the effects in one patient after he drank a special brand of coffee every Sunday morning. He was allergic to the particular coffee. He remained in a dark room in the bed with pain pills and water while rest of the family went to the Church. A man always had a gastrointestinal allergic attack on Sunday morning which often ended up in headaches. The cause was traced to eating a traditional pizza every Saturday night with his family. He was allergic to the tomato sauce on the pizza.

The time of day when the episodes occur is also of importance in determining the cause of an allergic manifestation. If it always occurs at night, it is quite likely that there is something in the bedroom that is aggravating the condition. It may be that the patient is sensitive to feathers in the pillow or comforter, wood cabinets, marble floors, carpets, side tables, end tables, bed sheets, pillows, pillow cases, detergents used in washing clothes, indoor plants, or shrubs, trees or grasses outside the patient's window.

Many patients react violently to house dust and suffer from headaches every time they clean the house. They could also react to different types of furniture, polishes, house plants, tap water and purified water and eventually lead to headaches.

The doctor should ask the patient to make a daily log of all the foods he/she is eating and all other daily activities. The ingredients in the food should be checked for possible allergens using NST. Certain common allergens like corn products, MSG (monosodium glutamate or Accent), citric acid, etc., are used in many food preparations.

Headaches are triggered by various food chemicals, food additives and gums used in many preparations: Acacia gum, xanthine gum, karaya gum, etc. Numerous gums are used in candy bars, yogurt, cream cheese, soft drinks, soy sauce, barbecue sauce, fast food products, macaroni and cheese, etc. Please refer to the list in Chapter 2 under *Ingestion*.

NAMBUDRIPAD'S TESTING TECHNIQUES (NTT)

NAET® uses many standard allopathic and kinesiological testing procedures to detect allergies. Some of the common ones are mentioned below.

1. HISTORY

A complete history of the patient is taken. A symptom survey form is given to the patient to record the level and type of discomfort he/she is suffering.

2. PHYSICAL EXAMINATION

Observation of the mental status, face, skin, eyes, color, posture, movements, gait, tongue, scars, wounds, marks, body secretions, etc.

3. VITAL SIGNS

Evaluation of blood pressure, pulse, skin temperature and palpable pains in the course of meridians, etc.

4. SRT (ELECTRO-DERMAL TEST-EDT)

Skin Resistance Test for the presence or absence of a suspected allergen is done through a computerized electrodermal testing device; differences in the meter reading are observed (the greater the difference, the stronger the allergy).

5. NST

Neuromuscular sensitivity testing (aka muscle response testing) is conducted to compare the strength of a predetermined muscle in the presence and absence of a suspected allergen. If the particular muscle (test muscle) weakens in the presence of an item, it signifies that the item is an allergen. If the muscle remains strong, the substance is not an allergen. More explanation on NST will be given in Chapter 5.

6. DYNAMOMETER TESTING

A hand-held dynamometer is used to measure finger strength (0-100 scale) in the presence and absence of a suspected allergen. The dynamometer is held with thumb and index finger and squeezed to make the reading needle swing between 0-100 scale. An initial base-line reading is observed first, then the allergen is held and another reading taken. The finger strength is compared in the presence of the allergen. If the second reading is more than the initial reading, there is no allergy. If the second reading is less than the initial reading, then there is an allergy.

7. EMF TEST (ELECTRO MAGNETIC FIELD TEST)

The electromagnetic component of the human energy field can be detected with simple muscle response testing. The pool of electromagnetic energy around an object or a person allows the energy exchange. The human field absorbs the energy from the nearby object and processes it through the network of nerve energy pathways. If the foreign energy field shares suitable charges with the human energy field, the human field absorbs the foreign energy for its advantage and becomes stronger. If the foreign energy field carries unsuitable charges, the human energy field causes repulsion of the foreign energy field. These types of reactions of the human field can be determined by testing an indicator muscle (specific muscle) before and after coming in contact with an allergen.

8. PULSE TEST

Pulse testing is another simple way of determining food allergy. This test was developed by Arthur Coca, M.D. in the 1950's. Research has shown that if you are allergic to something and you eat it, your pulse rate speeds up.

Step 1:   Establish your base-line pulse by counting radial pulse at the wrist for a full minute.

Step 2:   Put a small portion of the suspected allergen in the mouth, preferably under the tongue. Taste the substance for two minutes. Do not swallow any portion of it. The taste will send the signal to the brain, which will send a signal through the sympathetic nervous system to the rest of the body.

Step 3:   Retake the pulse with the allergen still in the mouth. An increase or decrease in pulse rate of 10% or more is considered an allergic reaction. The greater the degree of allergy, the greater the difference in the pulse rate. This test is useful to test food allergies. If you are allergic to very many foods, and if you consume a few allergens at the same time, it will be hard to detect the exact allergen causing the reaction just by this test.

9. NAET ROTATION DIET

After clearing the allergy to the basic NAET® allergens, the foods from the allergy-free list is consumed in a pre-selected order. Then use the question response test (ask questions while doing NST and the muscle weakness will be interpreted as "yes" answer, and a muscle strength will be interpreted as "no" answer. Every meal is selected from a non-allergic list according to the priority. This prevents overload of the particular food in the body and reduces unwanted allergic reactions and allergy-based disorders.

10. HOLD, SIT AND TEST

This is a simple procedure to test allergies. Place a small portion of the suspected allergen in a baby food jar or thin-glass jar, preferably with a lid, then the person will hold it in her/his palm, touching the jar with the fingertips of the same hand for 15 to 30 minutes. If the person is allergic to the item in the jar, he/she will begin to feel uneasy when holding the allergen in the palm, giving rise to various unpleasant symptoms. This testing procedure is described in detail in Chapter 6. When we treat patients who have a history of anaphylaxis to a particular item, we use this method after completing the required NAET® treatments and before the patient begins to use the item again.

If the patient was treated for a severe peanut allergy, (or milk, egg, wheat, fish, mushroom, etc.) after going through the required NAET® treatments to neutralize the peanut, the patient is allowed to sit and hold the peanuts in a glass jar every day for 30 minutes for three days to a week. If the patient does not show any symptoms of previous allergy, he/she will be allowed to hold a peanut in the hand without a bottle for three to five days, 30 minutes daily. If that does not produce any allergic reaction, then the patient will be allowed to put a small piece of nut in the mouth and hold it there for five to ten minutes every day for a few days. If that also does not produce any reaction, the patient will be allowed to eat a small piece of the nut and observe the reaction. Usually, by this time, the patient will be able to use the allergen confidently without fear. Check with your practitioner for more details.

11. ELISA/ACT

ELISA/ACT is distinctive in identifying reactions to all delayed or hidden immune reactions. This includes antibodies (functionally significant IgA, IgM, and IgG) as well as immune complexes and cell-mediated responses. Only a cell culture of all relevant lymphocyte (white cells with long life in circulation) types can give this information. ELISA/ACT is a highly sensitive cell response test which provides a specific fingerprint for each person by identifying substances, typically 6-20 items out of up to 340 that can be tested.

12. SCRATCH TEST

Western medical allergists generally depend on skin testing (scratch test, patch test, etc.), in which a very small amount of a suspected allergic substance is introduced into the person's skin through a scratch or an injection. The site of injection is observed for any reaction. If there is any reaction at the area of injection, the person is considered to be allergic to that substance. Each item has to be tested individually.

13. RADIOALLERGOSORBANT TEST (RAST)

The RAST measures IgE antibodies in serum and identifies specific allergens causing allergic reactions.

14. ELIMINATION DIET

The elimination diet, which was developed by Dr. Albert H. Rowe of Oakland, California, consists of a very limited diet that must be followed for a period long enough to determine whether or not any of the foods included in it are responsible for the allergic symptoms. The importance of adhering strictly to the diet during the diagnostic period is very crucial.

DIAGNOSIS OF HEADACHES

A detailed clinical history is the best diagnostic tool for any medical condition. It is extremely important for the patient, his/her parents or guardians to cooperate with the physician/NAET® specialist in giving all possible information to the doctor in order to obtain the best results. It is my hope that this chapter will help bring about a clearer understanding between NAET® specialists and their patients, because in order to obtain the most satisfactory results, both parties must work together as a team. Your NAET® specialist's office may ask you to complete a relevant questionnaire during your first appointment. It is important to provide as accurate a history as possible.

STEPS TO DIAGNOSE HEADACHES

Steps to establish the diagnosis of headache should consist of the following information about the patient.

1. General data sheet

2. Chief complaints

3. A detailed medical history

A detailed medical history should include the following information: presenting symptoms, pattern of symptoms, present medical history, frequency and severity of present symptoms (severity of the attacks, number of attacks by day, week, month, etc., number and frequency of hospitalizations, emergency room visits, response to medication, etc.), past medical history, personal health history, developmental history of the disease, prenatal history, growth and developmental history of the person, social history, behaviors, habits, occupation, hobbies, family history of headaches, precipitating or aggravating factors (effect of weather-change, exercise intolerance, change in living environment, job environment, etc.), short and long term goals expected from NAET® treatments.

4. Has the patient been seen by a neurologist or a specialist in diagnosing and treating headaches prior to this visit, if so, give the name and address of the physician. Information also should be collected about current pharmacological therapies, medications, herbs, nutritional supplements, dietary history, other therapies received in the past or currently receiving, information on radiolological and other diagnostic evaluations. Previous medical records from other medical facilities should be requested with the patient's consent if that is necessary to evaluate the patient's present health condition.

5. Impact of headaches on patient and family, assessment of patient's and family's perception of disease, information about family support or other support while going through the treatment also should be gathered.

6. The knowledge of the patient and family and/or caretakers on how to manage the headaches, exacerbations, and complications also should be noted.

7. Informed consent must be signed by the patient or gurdian giving permission to the NAET® specialist to provide the appropriate NAET® treatment using his/her expertise to help with the presenting condition.

GENERAL DATA SHEET

Gathering the patient's medical and related personal data is essential to understand the patient's background. This data sheet should contain the following information: age, gender, marital status, job situation, work address, home address, telephone numbers, other identifying information, and a next of kin to contact in emergency.

Review of personal data will help the NAET® specialist to understand the patient better: Is the patient a child/ under-age? A student? A mature adult? Employed or unemployed? Disabled due to illness? Capable of taking care of his/her needs, or dependent? Residential address, work address and job situation will help the NAET® sp to understand the living and working environments.

CHIEF COMPLAINTS

When did the headache start? The onset, intensity and duration.

If the patient is able, he/she is asked to describe the chief complaint in his/her own words. A patient suffering from a headache may present with the symptoms of throbbing or pulsating or dull head pain of moderate or severe intensity lasting from a few hours to days or more. The characteristics can include pain on one side of the head or both sides, unable to continue daily activities as usual, may accompany with depression, irritability, nausea, vomiting, visual disturbances, with aura or without aura. The intensity of the symptoms and duration of the headache will be varied.

[The reason for such NAET® symptom evaluation is as follows: The patient may have encountered a certain allergen that was capable of causing energy disturbances in the lung meridian, large intestine meridian, stomach meridian, spleen meridian, kidney meridian, urinary bladder meridian, liver meridian, gallbladder meridian and cental meridian, etc. (Read Chapter 5) giving rise to pathological symptoms evidenced by nausea, vomiting, depression, irritability, etc.]

PATTERN OF SYMPTOMS

The question should be asked about the pattern of frequency of occurrence of the attacks. Headaches may occur as seasonal or perennial, or both. The occurrence of headaches will be acute, chronic or episodic. The first onset of headache also varies largely in different people from childhood to any age depending on many factors. Some people suffer from headaches only during the day and some may suffer only at night. Some people get headaches upon waking up in the morning, some may get once a week and yet some may get only once a month or once a year. Some may get any time during the day and some get only at night or early morning and some are awakened in the middle of the night or early morning hours.We see all these variations.

[NAET® evaluation: There are many reasons for these huge variations in different manifestations in different people. Often the headache patient is sensitive to certain chemicals and other chemicals in the fabrics or encountered in everyday life. If symptoms occur only on specific days of the week, they are probably due to something contacted or eaten on that particular day. Although foods may be a contributing factor, if the symptoms occur only at specific times of the year, the cause most likely is due to something that is predominant around the patient at that time; for example: a particular grass pollen or flower pollen in the air or may be the dust or wind during the windy season. Man has a natural tolerance for food that prevents the manifestation of headache until one saturates the body with the particular allergic food or until the newly encountered chemical or substance adds sufficient allergens to throw the body into an imbalance. The time of day when the attacks occur is also of importance in determining the cause of headache. If it always occurs before mealtime, low blood sugar may be a possible cause. If it occurs after meals, an allergy to something in the meal should be suspected. If it occurs regularly at bedtime, the toothbrush, toothpaste, mouth wash, makeup remover, night cream, night attire, etc., may be suspected. If it occurs regularly at night, it is quite likely that there is something in the bedroom that is aggravating the condition. It may be that the patient is sensitive to: feathers in the pillow, comforter, bed frame, mattress, wood cabinets, marble floors, carpets, side tables, end tables, bed sheets, pillows, pillow cases, detergents used in washing clothes, indoor plants, shrubs, trees, bed partner (an allergy to people), or grasses outside the patient's window.

One of my 67-year old female patients suffered from severe migraine-type headaches, twice a week for many years. She woke up always with headaches in the morning and the pain continued for rest of the day or more even if she took strong prescription medication. She was found to be allergic to her bean sprout-salad she ate so faithfully twice a week for years ever since she was told by an Eastern herbal doctor that eating bean sprouts twice a week could maintain her youthfullness for a long time. It sure helped her to maintain her youthfullness. She looked at least ten years younger than her actual age. She was also found to be allergic to many amino acids. Soon she was desensitized for the bean sprouts, and all necessary individual amino acids through

Say Good-bye to Headaches

NAET. Now she can enjoy the bean sprouts without triggering headaches and continue to maintain the youthfullness.

The cause of disease can, at first, appear random. One young patient experienced regular attacks of headaches after his physical education classes at school. This young man was found to be allergic to exercise. He was allergic to endorphin, a brain chemical produced during exercise.

Another young man complained of headaches at about 10:00 am almost daily. He had math classes between 9:00 to 10:00 AM. He attributed his headaches to the dislike he had towards his math class and the teacher. He did not have headaches during the weekends and Holidays. When we evaluated him in our office, it was revealed that he was allergic to the cinnamon toast cereal he had daily in the morning before he went to school. About two hours after he ate the cereal, he got the headaches, which also happened to be the math class that he didn't quite like. During weekends and holidays, his mother prepared pancakes for him so he never ate the cinnamon toast ceral for breakfast. He was desensitized for the cinnamon and the cereal, ever since he hasn't had his usual migraines.

A boy always developed a severe headache while doing his home work at home. When he completed the work he would take a couple of pain pills and go to bed. He would be free of headaches until the following evening when he begins the homework. He was found to be allergic to the wooden desk where he did his homwork. He was asked to bring a small sample of his desk (a small sample of wood shaving from inside part of the desk will make a good sample), and desensitized him for it. He stopped having headaches ever since.

A young 7-year-old boy complained of frequent frontal headaches whenever he colored his books. He was allergic to crayons and the colors affected his stomach meridians.

A 44-year-old female suffered from severe frequent headaches and she was found to be allergic to the serotonin found in the turkcy. She ate turkey frequently for lunch to keep the calories down. Turkey is a good source of serotonin, one of the brain enzymes that is necessary for normal brain functions. She was desensitized for the serotonin and turkey. Since then she hasn't had her usual headaches even though she ate turkey regularly.

Another woman with frequent headaches was found to be allergic to a particular jacket she used frquently. She was advised to put the jacket away for a couple of weeks. She did not have headaches during that time. Then she was asked to wear it again on for two days off for two days for a couple of weeks. Each time she used the jacket, her headaches returned within an hour of wearing it and did not have any headache on the days when she did not use it. She tried this game for a month. Then she returned to office with her research data. It was amazing to see the result. Then she was desensitized for the material on the jacket, lining, and name tag, and she became free of her headaches.

No one has any explanation to why certain bodies react towards some things in certain way. An item may be absolutely harmless to one person and completely disastrous to the sensitive person.

PRESENT HISTORY

A careful medical history, and appropriate NTTs (Nambudripad's Testing Techniques include: Physical examination, kinesiological tests and other relevant diagnostic studies) will provide the information needed to ensure a correct diagnosis of headache. Some typical preliminary questions should include the following format of questioning.

When did your or your child's first symptom of headache occur?

Did you notice your or your child's headache as a child, or during adolescence?

Did it occur after going through a certain procedure? For example, did it occur for the first time after a dental procedure, like applying braces or filling a cavity?

Did it happen after the first antibiotic treatment?

Did it happen after installing a water filter?

Did it happen after you started sleeping on a waterbed?

Did it happen after receiving a birthday present? A tricycle, a pearl necklace, a cotton summer dress? A hair dryer?

Did it begin after starting on a new weight loss diet?

Did it begin after started to take a new vitamin supplement?

Did it occur after a booster dose of immunization?

Did it happen after putting in a lawn?

Did it happen after putting in a flower bed?

Did it happen after putting in a vegetable garden?

Did it happen after picking fruits from a tree?

Did it happen after working in the vegetable or fruit garden?

Did it happen after putting fertilizer on the plants?

Did it happen after spraying insecticides or pesticides to the plants in your garden?

Did it happen after spraying insecticides or pesticides to the plants in your neighborhood by the city workers?

Did it happen after eating vegetables and fruits from your garden?

Did it happen after you took a walk in the park?

Did your headache begin after taking a long drive in the new automobile?

Did your headache begin after you received or bought that beautiful gold necklace?

Next, the doctor will want to know the circumstances surrounding and/or immediately preceding the first symptoms. Typical questions will include:

Did you change your or the child's diet or put him/her on a special diet?

Did you or he/she eat something that hadn't been eaten recently, perhaps for two or three months?

Did you eat or feed your child one type of food repeatedly, say, every day?

Did the headache follow an illness, (fever, bronchitis, cough, chicken pox, strept-throat) or any medication for such an illness?

Did your headache follow some other illness such as influenza, pneumonia, a viral infection, bacterial infection, parasitic infestation, or a treatment program for any of these?

Did your headache follow a major operation?

Did the headache begin after your vacation to an island, to another country?

Did the headache begin after camping in a cold, damp, camp ground?

Did the headache begin after an earthquake?

Did the headache begin after living through a tornado?

Did your headache begin after wearing dry-cleaned clothes?

Did your headache begin after walking in the rain?

Did your headache begin after spraying pesticides in your neighborhood? Or walking in the park where the pesticide was sprayed earlier?

Did your headache begin after eating a special food?

Did your headache begin after using a special chemical to clean your carpet?

Did your headache begin after getting a new car?

Did your headache begin after bringing new furniture into the house?

Did your headache begin after visiting a cigarette-smoke-filled casino?

Did your headache begin after taking a course of antibiotics?

Did your headache begin after starting a new vitamin supplement?

Did your headache begin after going through a detoxification program?

Did your headache begin after receiving other therapy, say for arthritis? Kidney dialysis? Blood transfusion? Dental work?

Did your headache begin after an auto accident? Any other accident?

Did your headache begin after receiving traumatic news?

Did your headache begin after starting a new exercise program?

Did your headache begin with any emotional trauma, like the house burning down during a wild fire, etc?

Did your headache begin after the loss of a loved one?

Did your headache begin after the loss of a pet?

Did your headache begin after the loss of a toy?

Did your headache begin with sadness?

Did your headache begin with grief?

Did your headache begin with guilt?

Did your headache begin with frustration? Embarrassment? Shame?

Did your headache begin with any stress, like loss of job, divorce, etc?

Any one of these factors can be responsible for triggering a headache or precipitate the noticeable symptoms of headache condition. Therefore, it is very important for an NAET® practitioner/doctor to obtain full and accurate answers when taking the patient's medical history.

PRESENT SYMPTOMS

The NAET® specialist will gather information about the frequency of headaches and the severity of the attacks in the patient's own words.

How often do you get headaches? _____

Daily_____Any particular time of the day? _____

Every other day_____Once a week _____

Once a month _____

Once a year _____

How long does an attack last? _____

Do you take any medication?   Yes [ ]   No [ ]

If you marked yes, please list your medications _____

_____

Do you get relief after medication?   Yes [ ]   No [ ]

If so within how many minutes? _____

Do you go to the emergency room to get relief? Yes [ ] No [ ]

How many times have you received emergency care for your headaches during this week? _____

Last month?_____

Last 3 months? _____

Last 6 months? _____

Last 12 months_____

The information should be obtained in the following areas:

The charateristics of the headaches:

Headache on the forehead   Yes [ ] No [ ]

Headaches on the side(s) of the head   Yes [ ] No [ ]

Headaches on the top of the head   Yes [ ] No [ ]

Headaches on the back of the head   Yes [ ] No [ ]

After Meals   Yes [ ] No [ ]

Before Meals   Yes [ ] No [ ]

After using any special products

(chewing gum, perfume,etc.)   Yes [ ] No [ ]

Nature of the pain throbing or pulsationg   Yes [ ] No [ ]

Sensation of a tight band around the head   Yes [ ] No [ ]

Excrutiating, sudden headaches   Yes [ ] No [ ]

Headaches with aura   Yes [ ] No [ ]

Headaches without aura   Yes [ ] No [ ]

Headaches with nausea, vomiting, etc.   Yes [ ] No [ ]

After certain activities _____

If so, list the activity_____.

OTHER FACTORS CAUSING HEADACHES

- Viral or bacterial infection.
- Sinusitis, hay-fever, or rhinitis.
- Nasal polyp or gastroesophageal reflex disorders
- Enlarged glands, lymph nodes, growth, tumors and cancers.
- Santa Ana wind, moving to new living quarters, change of living environment, job situation, between jobs, hor-

monal changes, function.

- Weather changes
- Other health problems and medication taking for such conditions.
- Acquired a pet
- Food or drug sensitivity and allergies.

PAST MEDICAL HISTORY

It is important to review the past medical history. History of development of headaches, previous treatments, age of first onset, frequency of occurrences, number of hospital admissions, emergency room visits, etc. should be obtained. History of any previous accidents, infections, diseases, taking any special medications, hormone supplements, vitamin supplements, special diets, special therapies, bought anything new prior to beginning the headaches, any special procedures done, new relationships, acqured a pet, or had any unusual or upsetting emotional event(s).

If the patient has done any previous diagnosistic studies, or treatment at another facility, copies of the reports, treatment records, medication history, and progress reports from them should be requested. Also a record of any history of allergic symptoms in the patient should be made. The patient will be asked if he/she ever suffered from arthritis, asthma, hay-fever, rhinitis, sinusitis, frequent lung infections, constipation, hives, eczema, food sensitivities, dyspepsia, indigestion, joint pains, mood swings, reacted to a serum injection (such as tetanus antitoxin, DPT), bothered by weather changes, humidity, suffered from headaches in warm weather, in high altitudes, bothered by extreme weathers like cold or heat, throat closing-like sensation with ice cream or any other foods, or any other conditions where an allergy might have been a contributing factor for the headaches.

PERSONAL HEALTH HISTORY

Characteristics of home including age of the home, location, cooling and heating system, wood burning stove, humidifier, carpeting over concrete, presence of molds, or mildew, characteristics of rooms where patient spends time: e.g., bedroom, and living room with attention to bedding, floor covering, stuffed furniture, picture frames, fireplace, indoor plants, animals, outdoor plants, any vines, trees, shrubs growing near the bedroom window, any unclean old spa or swimming pool near the bedroom, or any collection of junk outside the bedroom causing molds and mildew to grow. Also questions about any smell in or around the house should be asked. Smells from cooking, baking, coffee brewing, herbal concoctions, and other smells including perfume, aftershave lotion, shampoo, body lotion, smoking (patient and others in home or day care, workplace, and school surroundings) etc. which can trigger headaches in some people.

Other impeding factors such as peer pressure, fear from different sorts, substance abuse, gang involvements, cult involvements, etc. may trigger headaches in some people.

Questions also should be asked about the level of education completed, past or present employment (if employed, characteristics of work environment), family support, social support, or other support.

DEVELOPMENTAL HISTORY OF THE DISEASE

History of early life and developmental information through the years should be obtained if available. Many patients react violently to house dust, different types of furniture, polishes, house plants, tap water and purified water. Most of the city water suppliers change the water chemicals once or twice a year. People with chemical allergies may get headaches if they inhale or ingest the same chemicals over and over for a period of time. Some patients who live near any chemical factories, factories that generate pesticides, insecticides, radioactive materials, living near high voltage electric circuits, environmental and chemical waste dumping areas, refuse dumps, cotton fields, gradually develop headaches over a period of time due to overexposure to the toxins and toxic wastes. If a person is allergic to radiation (computer, television, X-ray radiation, microwave radiation, etc.), eventually he/she can develop headaches. People living near a park (exposure to pesticides), working in a furniture factory (exposure to pesticides and heavy metals, PBDE - polybrominated diphenyl -a fire retardant chemical used in furniture making), working in a swimming pool supply area, working with lead, silica, etc., working in pest control companies, working in fabric companies, people in sewing business are prone to get headaches. If the patient is a child, it is very important to get the complete prenatal history, growth and developnmental history.

PRENATAL HISTORY

Information on all these issues: socio-economic factors; exposures to substance abuse, heavy metal poisoning, coffee, alcohol, chemical toxins, carbon monoxide poisoning, bacterial toxins; emotional traumas during fetal development or later years; birth records including birth weight and APGAR scores.

GROWTH AND DEVELOPMENTAL HISTORY

ILLNESSES DURING EARLY INFANCY

Presence of any of these symptoms in infancy or childhood will confirm the inherited allergic tendency even though it was not manifested as asthma at that time. Mark it with a check in the appropriate column.

[ ]   Colic

[ ]   Constipation

[ ]   Diarrhea

[ ]   Feeding problem

[ ]   Excessive vomiting

[ ]   Excessive white coating on the tongue

[ ]   Excessive crying

[ ]   Poor sleep

[ ]   Disturbed sleep

[ ]   Frequent ear infection

[ ]   Frequent fever

[ ]   Immunizations

[ ]   Response to the immunizations

[ ]   Common childhood diseases like measles, chickenpox, mumps, strep-throat, etc.

[ ]   Any other unusual events (fire in the house, accidents, earthquakes, smoke inhalation, carbon monoxide poisoning, death in the family, a new pet, etc).

DEVELOPMENTAL MILESTONES

Mark with a check in the appropriate column. Write the age, year, frequency, or number of times, if applicable.

AGE OF THE CHILD

[ ]   Walked alone————————————

[ ]   Talked —————————————

[ ]   Toilet trained for bladder
      and bowel ————————————

[ ]   Enrolled in school ——————————

MEDICAL HISTORY OF EARLY LIFE

[ ]   Surgeries————————

[ ]   Hospitalizations ——————

[ ]   Diseases ————————

[ ]   Allergies ————————

[ ]   Frequent colds ——————

[ ]   Fever ————————

[ ]   Ear infections ——————

[ ]   Asthma ————————

[ ]   Hives ————————

[ ]   Bronchitis ————————

[ ]   Pneumonia ———————

[ ]   Seizures ————————

[ ]   Sinusitis ————————

[ ]   Headaches ———————

[ ]   Vomiting ————————

[ ]   Diarrhea ————————

[ ]   Current medication —————

[ ]   Any reaction to medication ———

[ ]   Antibiotics and drugs taken ———

[ ]   Parasitic infestation —————

[ ]   Visited other countries —————

SOCIAL HISTORY

Learning: Grades at school, interaction between friends and teachers, interaction between family members, activities at school, phobias, and problems with discipline. (A child may not yet manifest with obvious headache symptoms, but allergies to things in his/her environment can cause the child have problems in any of these areas. Eventually such allergies can manifest in headaches).

Behaviors: Cooperative, uncooperative, disruptive and/or aggressive behaviors; overactive, restless, inattentive, day dreams; uncooperative with his/her peers and adults; incomplete or sloppy work (These also could be due to allergies to food additives and other chemicals).

Habits: Obsession, compulsion, frequent clearing of the throat, itching and picking nose, vomiting after meals, temper tantrums, depression, quietness, remain isolated and not playing with others, clinging to mother all the time (feelings of insecurity), restless leg syndrome (an allergy to food or something in the bed), unusual fears and fatigue.

Hobbies: Reading, golfing, tennis, walking in the park, horseback riding, painting, etc.

Occupation: Students, writers, lawyers, doctors, bakers, cooks, managers in different areas, store keepers, beauticians, cleaners, gardeners, teachers, painters, road workers, field workers, factory workers, engineers, drivers, entertainers, etc.

No job is exempted from getting exposed to dangerous allergens. Potential allergens are hiding in unexpected places and any one of them can trigger a headache in a sensitive person. Avoiding the allergen is not a permanent solution. Running away from a problem will not help us to solve the problem. One needs to face the problem and eliminate it. NAET® treatments can eliminate the problems permanently.

FAMILY HISTORY

The medical history of the immediate relatives, mother, father, and siblings should be noted. The questions should be asked about history of arthritis, asthma, allergy, sinusitis, rhinitis, sinus surgeries, or nasal polyps in patient's immediate relatives. The same questions are asked about the patient's non-immediate relatives: grandparents, aunts, uncles, brothers, sisters, cousins. A tendency to get sick or have allergies or headaches is not always inherited directly from the parents. It may skip generations or manifest in nieces or nephews rather than in direct descendants.

The inquiry should include not only about headaches, but other allergy-related health disorders like alcoholism, autoimmune disorders, drug abuse, smoking, eating disorders, addictive behaviors, mental disorders, other health disorders. The careful NAET® specialist will also determine whether or not diseases such as tuberculosis, cancer, heart disease, diabetes, hypoglycemia, rheumatic or glandular disorders exist, or have ever occurred in the patient's family history.

All of these facts help give the NAET® specialist a complete picture of the hereditary characteristics of the patient. An allergy may be manifested differently in different people, even if it is familial. For example, parents may have had cancer or rheumatism, but the child can manifest that inheritance as headaches.

COMPLICATING FACTORS

A single allergen, or a group of allergens, or an incident may have triggered the headache in a patient. But it usually does not end there. More allergens from the environment will begin to affect the weakened immune system of the victim. He/she may have been allergic to a large group of substances in the surroundings but until an allergen triggered a major reaction, others were kept under control by the body's natural defense. When the first major allergen sets forth the initiative, a chain reaction will begin with all other allergens causing cascades of reactions creating more complication for the sufferer. Such people can suffer from headaches many times a week in varying degrees and intensities, taking a long time to respond to any medication or therapy. Aggravating factors should be avoided or the reaction between the body and the allergens should be eliminated (via NAET® treatments) before they can show any response to the medication or therapy. Some of the commonly seen allergens which can act like triggers can be seen in the following lists.

DO THE SYMPTOMS OCCUR OR WORSEN:

AFTER INHALING SUBSTANCES

Inhaling pollens while walking in the park when the pollen count is high; inhaling after-shave lotions, airborne chemicals, benzene, body lotions, body soap, chemical smells from city water, cigarette smoke, cleansing agents, colognes, cooking smells, cosmetic products, cut grass smell, dental materials, detergents, diesel, dust, exhausts, fabric softeners, fertilizers, fireplace smoke, flowers, food seasoning smell, formaldehyde, frying food smell, fungicides, gasoline, hair products, hair sprays, herbal supplements, herbicides, hospital supplies (smell from oxygen tubes, rubber or plastic catheters, surgical instruments, surgical sutures, hospital cleaning agents, disinfectants, anesthetics, drugs), house cleaning chemicals, house dust, and dust mites, hydrocarbons, insects (cockroach, bee, fly, flea, ants, etc.), insecticide sprays, laboratory chemicals, leather smell, massage oils, molds and mildews, fungus, new car smell, newspaper ink, newspaper, paper products, outdoor allergens (tree pollens, trees, shrubs, weeds, flowers, grass, fibers floating in the air from cotton pods when they mature before picking them from the trees, lint wastage from cotton mills and other fabric mills, fumes from chemical factories, silica dust from silica factory, radioactive waste or fallout from the storage or factory, paint fumes, etc.), perfumes, personal protective equipment (latex gloves, masks), pesticides, plastic products, polishes, prescription drugs, shampoo, smell from animals and animal products, smell from cat litter, smell from coffee brewing, smell from candle burning, smell from food, smell from popcorn, smell from paint fumes, smell from soiled baby-diaper, smell of body secretions (saliva, semen, vaginal discharge, sputum, sweat, bad breath, menstrual blood, stool, urine, body odor), smell from room fresheners, soap, sugar cane burning smoke, wild fire burning smoke, synthetic fabrics, tobacco smoke, varnishes, vitamins, wood burning smoke, wood furniture, wood polish.

AFTER INGESTING ANY MEAL

Alcoholic drinks, antibiotics (in meat, milk, other products), artificial food coloring, beans, bell pepper, beverages, cactus, carob, chewing gums, chicken, chocolate, cinnamon, condiments, cooked food, cooking sprays, corn, dried fruits, drinking water, drinks, drugs (aspirin, beta-blockers, nonsteroidal anti-inflammatory drugs, cardiac, analgesics, topicals, and others), egg plant, eggs, fish, food additives, food preservatives, fruits, garlic, grains, grapes, hormone supplements, meat, medication, melons, mushroom, nutmeg, nuts, onion, pain relieving medication, pineapple, potato, prenatal vitamins, prepackaged food, protein drinks, rain water, raisins, salt, sea salt, sea water, soy products, special diets, spices, sugar, sulfites, thyroid medication, tomato, uncooked food, vegetables, vitamins, weight loss diets, water chemicals, water filter salts, wheat, and yeast.

AFTER CONTACTING CERTAIN SUBSTANCES

Acetate, acrylic, animal dander, animal epithelial, bathroom slippers, bed linen, animals and animals with fur or feathers, bed room furniture, books, carpets, ceramic cups, ceramic tiles, chair, cleaning chemicals, cockroach, coloring books, coloring equipments, cooking pans, cotton fabrics, crayons, crib toys, curtains, dental equipment, dental filling materials, dentures, dining table, dishwashing soap, down comforter, drapes, elastics, electronic toys, exercising equipments, feather pillows, hair brush, hair dryer, heavy metals, highlighters, house plants in the bed room, house-dust mites, interior decorating materials, jewelry, kitchen cleaning materials like scrubbers, latex products, liquid paper, mattress, mercury, mouth wash, night blooming plants if the window is left open, night wear clothes, office products, other fabrics, paintings, pencils, pens, personal hygiene products, pillows, plastic sheets, plastic toys, prosthesis, pajama, reading books, remote control for the TV, rubber, sanitary napkins, school bag, school desk, school work material, shoe, silverware, socks, stuffed toys, table cloth, table mat, tampons, tap water, teflon coating on the pans, tennis ball, tennis racket, the night air, toothbrush, toothpaste, underwear, upholstered furniture, wall paint, wall picture, wall poster, water bed, work material, and wristwatch.

AFTER INJECTING ANYTHING INTO THE BODY

Allergy shots, insulin shots, vitamin shots, hormone shots, vaccinations, immunizations, insect bites, mosquito bites, bee stings, stung by corals, shellfish, sea urchins, dog bites, cat scratches, animal bites of other sources, bitten by ticks, fleas, flies, ants, etc.

AFTER CONTACTING INFECTIOUS AGENTS

After exposure to virus, bacteria, parasite, either exposed through eating uncooked or spoiled foods or lived in closed contact with people with viral, bacterial infections, parasitical infestation, molds, mildews, fungi, decayed materials, or suffering from other contagious diseases. Sometimes infections can spread by contacting the materials handled by the suffering person: utensils, silverware, body secretions, sharing the same toilet, bath towels, etc.

AFTER EXPOSURE TO EXTREME WEATHER CONDITIONS

Heat, cold, playing in the snow, dryness, dampness, humid conditions, fog, wind, damp-heat, damp-cold, draughts, cold air from air conditioner, etc.

AFTER EXPOSURE TO OCCUPATIONAL HAZARDS

Tobacco smoke, strong odors, air pollutants, occupational chemicals, dusts particles, cleaning chemicals, noises, airplane fuel or exhaust, airplane noises, vapors and gases.

AFTER EXPERIENCING EMOTIONAL TRAUMAS

After facing events leading to excessive laughing, excessive crying, sadness, grief, frustration, betrayal, depression, aggression, fear, anger, diagnosed with an unexpected new disease such as cancer, diagnostic testing procedures, surgery, changing homes, places, moving to another country, new friends, new life experiences, new additions to the family by birth or marriage, financial loss, human loss, material loss, post traumatic stress disorders, etc.

SUDDEN CHANGE IN LIVING ENVIRONMENTS

Molds, mildews, fungi, decayed materials in the new environments, moving home, buying new home, renovation or construction of the home, vacation, changing jobs, changing states, country, new life-style, changing schools, starting a new school, starting a new career, starting a new life, etc.

WHEN GOING THROUGH HORMONAL CHANGES

Changes in the status of menses, pregnancy, delivery, thyroid imbalances, pituitary imbalances, people who suffer from gastroesophageal reflex disorders, congestive heart failure, heart diseases, kidney disorders, people on dialysis, etc.

DURING OR AFTER EXERCISE

During exercise, production of endorphins, enkaphalins, neurotransmitters, and certain hormones like pheromones, etc., are stimulated. If the patient is allergic to these secretions they can trigger headaches in sensitive people. Some people get sinus congestion, and pressure on the top of the head during sexual intimacy. That is because the patient may be allergic to pheromones produced by the body during sexual intimacy.

Role of NAET® Specialist

1. Short Term Goal of NAET® for Headaches

II. Long Term Goals of NAET® for Headache

I. Short Term Goal of NAET® for Headaches

A. Prevent Occurrences of Headaches

Prevent headaches by treating the patient for NAET® basic allergens. Two or three times a week treatment is advised initially in order to complete the treatment on the first 20 NAET® basic allergens in order to provide the patient some early relief of headaches.

Eighty percent of people with headaches diminish their symptoms and reduce the need for much medications by the time they successfully complete treatments for 20-30 NAET® basic groups of allergens.

B. Improve Quality of Life

1. Avoid all known allergens until treated.

2. Continue all medications and therapies as prescribed.

3. Increase the activity as tolerated.

II. Long Term Goals of NAET for Headaches

1.   Maintain normal activity levels.

3.   Prevent recurrent headaches

4.   Prevent exacerbations of headaches.

5.   Minimize emergency room visits and hospitalizations.

6.   Improve the quality of life.

7.   Educate the patient, family or caretakers/assistants about NAET® home testing procedures to detect the triggers so that the triggers can be avoided.

1. Maintain Regular Health Record

Patient should be referred to a qualified neurologist for consultation if the patient is not seeing one already and co-management with pharmacotherapy in the initial stages of headaches and to maintain complete health record including the results of blood chemistries. It is very important to encourage the patient to keep his/her headaches under control while reciving NAET® so that NAET® treatments can be performed without any disturbances. If the symptoms are kept under control, NAET® works better. In milder cases, herbs and nutritional supplements might help control the headaches while going through NAET® treatments. Severe cases must seek appropriate pharmacotherapy to keep the symptoms under control until the allergens are treated and eliminated from your life.

2.   Maintaining Normal Activity Levels

1. Treat all known allergens through NAET®.

2. Maintain a daily treatment log or journal.

3. Prevent Recurrent Headaches

A. The patient should be taught NAET® self-testing.

B. The patient should be taught NAET® headaches reducing points and teach them to use at the first sign of headache.

4. Prevent Exacerbations of Headaches

The patient should be taught NAET® self-balancing, and adivise them to do them daily, twice a day, until they are free of headaches

5. Minimize E.R.visits or Hospitalizations

A. The patient should learn the acupressure emergency

help points.

B. The patient should carry epi-pen and antihistamines all the time and never hesitate to use them when they are needed.

C. The patient should call 911 or seek emergency help immediately when needed in any acute situation.

6. Improve the Long-term Quality of Life

A. The patient should avoid all known allergens until treated with NAET®.

B. Nutritional evaluation and supplementation to maintain adequate nutrition.

C. Follow-up with the NAET® specialist regularly for the treatments until the known allergens are treated.

D. After treating for all known allergens, continue follow-up visits with the NAET® specialist on the following schedule:

1. Once a month for three months, once in three months for the first year, once in six months for the second year, and then once a year.

2. Follow-up with the neurologist: Once in six months for five years for complete evaluation oof the system. Then yearly check up should be enough provided you do not get any more episodes of headaches.

7. Educate the patient and family

A. The family and caretakers should help the patient avoid the item from the patient's list of detected allergens until the patient is treated for them.

B. The family should be taught NAET® self-testing.

C. The family should be taught NAET® headache reducing points and teach them to use at the first sign of head pain.

SELF-TESTING

The NAET® sp should teach the patient self-testing using "O" Ring test, Finger-on-finger test, and Dynamometer testing. Family or the helper should also learn how to test for allergies using Neuro Muscular Sensitivity Testing.

SELF-BALANCING

Acupressure self-balancing techniques are given with illustration in Chapter 6 for headaches. More acupressure therapeutic points for various disorders can be learnt from my book, "Living Pain Free" and can be purchased from www.amazon.com or from NAET® website. The patient can easily learn to balance his/her body using these pressure points. According to Oriental medical theory, when the body is maintained at perfect balance, diseases or allergic reactions do not happen. The patient is encouraged to self-balance twice a day, upon awakening and before going to bed. The family or helper can also be taught to balance the patient using these headache-reducing acuhelp points.

ACUPRESSURE EMERGENCY HELP POINTS

Acupressure emergency help points are given with illustration in Chapter 6. Knowing how to use these Oriental medicine Cardio Pulmonary Resuscitation (CPR) points can help you overcome immediate emergencies and help you stay awake and alive until help arrives or until you are able to call for help or reach the nearest emergency room. The family or helper could also learn how to use these acupressure emergency resuscitation points.

ADVICE TO THE FAMILY

NAET® specialist should meet with the patient's family and caretakers or assistants in his/her care and educate them about the importance of undrstanding the signs, and symptoms of headaches and the possibility of sudden exacerbations if the patient comes in contact with any allergen. Family and caretakers should be taught to avoid the allergens from the patient's list of detected allergens until the patient is treated for them when the patient is nearby. If someone eats the allergen around the patient, he/she can react to it and trigger headache. So other family members should avoid the patient's allergens from being eaten or used when the patient is nearby. Family members need to be aware of the impact of the patient's sickness on the family, if he/she gets a sudden severe headache and if he/she needs to go to the emergency room or hospital. If they learn to test and not to expose the patient to known allergens, they can avoid unwanted emergencies.

NUTRITIONAL EVALUATION

When someone has allergies to basic everyday foods, he/she may not be absorbing the essential nutritients from the daily food. This malabsorption creates a huge nutritional deficiency in the patient. The NAET® Basic treatments are made up of essential nutrients from one's daily diet. More detailed explanation about NAET® Basic treatments is given in Chapter 6. After eliminating the allergy, the essential nutrients should be supplemented for faster recovery.

EVALUATION OF ACTIVITY

Importance of moderate amount of exercise cannot be stressed enough. Exercise is necessary to help improve the circulation in order to distribute the nutrients to different parts of the body. Improved circulation will also help eliminate the toxins from the body. Encourage the patient to add some mild exercise plan into the daily agenda.

FOLLOW-UP WITH NAET®

Follow-up with your NAET® specialist regularly for treatments until the known allergens are treated and desensitized. The NAET® Guidebook (available at www.naet.com or www.amazon.com) is a very important and useful handbook to help you successfully complete the NAET® treatments. After treating for all known allergens, continue follow-up visits with your NAET specialist with the following schedule: Once a month for three months, once in three months for the first year, once in six months for the second year, and then onwards once a year or as and when the need arises.

Patient should continue to maintain the daily log of foods eaten, foods not eaten but prepared by the patient, and any problems encountered while cooking or eating. Any unusual events happened to physical health or emotional health, any trips made to other cities, had to live through any disasters like earthquakes, tornado, flood, fire disaster, smoke inhalation, etc. should be recorded in the log and brought to the NAET® sp at each visit. The NAET® sp will evaluate your physical and emotional responses to the events and if needed he/she will provide NAET® to eliminate the effects of the trauma(s).

FOLLOW-UP WITH THE NEUROLOGIST

Patient should be seen by a Neurologist for regular evaluation as often as needed during the treatment phase. After completing the NAET® program, patient should visit neurologist one in six months for five years for complete evaluation. Patient should have a complete examination of all systems every six months to ensure the safety of the patient's health. Patient should refill the prescription for analgesics and carry with them always at least for five years after completing NAET® program. If the patient never had another headache episode in five years following the completion of NAET® treatment program, then the patient can discuss with his/her neurologist regarding the need for further carrying the analgesics with him/her all the time. NAET® specialist will not help you make that decision.

CHAPTER 4

Symptoms of Meridians

An allergy means an altered reactivity. Reactions and after-effects can be measured using various standard medical diagnostic tests. Energy medicine has also developed various devices to measure the reactions. Oriental medicine has used "Medical I Ching" since 3,322 BC. Another simple way to test one's body is through simple, kinesiological neuromuscular sensitivity testing (NST) procedures (Chapter 5). It is an easy procedure for a person to evaluate his/her progress.

Study of the acupuncture meridians is helpful to understand NST and how it works. All living beings have energy meridians and nerve energy circulates through these merdians throughout the day and night. If one learns to identify abnormal symptoms connected with acupuncture meridians, detection of the causative agents will be easier. The pathological functions of the twelve major acupuncture meridians, and their functions are described in the next few pages.

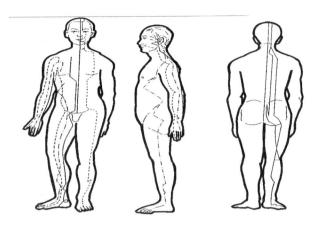

**ENERGY FLOW THROUGH 12 MERIDIANS
FIGURE 4-1**

NORMAL ENERGY FLOW

Lung--> Large Intestine--> Stomach-->Spleen--> Heart--> Small Intestine-->Urinary Bladder--> Kidney--> Pericardium-->Triple Warmer--> Gall Bladder--> Liver->Lung

THE LUNG MERIDIAN (LU)

Energy disturbance in the lung meridian affecting physical and physiological levels can give rise to the following symptoms:

Asthma between 3-5 a.m.
Atopic dermatitis
Bronchiectasis
Bronchitis
Burning in the eyes, & nostrils
Cardiac asthma
Chest congestion & cough
Coughing up blood
Cradle cap
Dry mouth, skin, throat
Emaciated look
Emphysema
Fever with chills
Frequent flu-like symptoms
General body ache with burning
    sensation
Generalized hives
Hair loss
Hair thinning
Hay-fever
Headache between eyes
Inability to sleep after 3 a.m.
Infantile eczema
Infection in the respiratory tract
Itching of the body, scalp, nose
Lack of desire to talk
Lack or excessive of perspiration
Laryngitis and pharyngitis
Low voice
Moles
Morning fatigue
Mucus in the throat
Nasal congestion or runny nose

Night sweats
Nose bleed
Pain between third and fourth
    thoracic vertebrae
Pain in the chest and intercostal
    muscles
Pain in the eyes
Pain in the first interphalangeal
    joint and thumb
Pain in the upper arms and back
Pain in the upper first and second
    cuspids (tooth)
Pleurisy
Pneumonia
Poor growth of nails and hair
Postnasal drip
Red cheeks and eyes
Restlessness between
    3 to 5 a.m.
Scaly and rough skin
Sinus headaches and infection
Skin rashes
Skin tags
Sneezing
Sore throat
Stuffy nose
Swollen cervical glands
Swollen throat
Tenosynovitis
Thick yellow discharge in case of
bacterial infection
Thin or thick white discharge in
    case of viral infection

Say Good-bye to Headaches

Energy disturbance in the lung meridian affecting the cellular level. When one fails to cry, when one feels deep sorrow, sadness will settle in the lungs and eventually cause various lung disorders

Apologizing
Comparing self with others
Contempt
Dejection
Depression
Despair
False pride
Grief or sadness.
Highly sensitive emotionally
Hopelessness
Intolerance

Likes to humiliate others
Loneliness
Low self-esteem
Meanness
Melancholy
Over demanding
Over sympathy
Prejudice
Seeking approval from others
Self pity
Weeping Frequently

Essential Nutrients to Strengthen the Lung Meridian

Clear water
Proteins
Vitamin A
Vitamin C
Bioflavonoid
Cinnamon
Essential fatty acids
Onions
Garlic

B-vitamins (especially B$_2$)
Citrus fruits
Green peppers
Black peppers
Rice

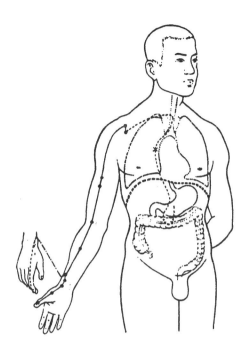

FIGURE 4-1

THE LUNG MERIDIAN (LU)

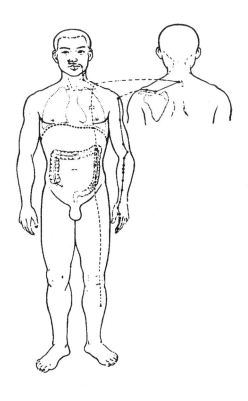

FIGURE 4-2

THE LARGE INTESTINE MERIDIAN (LI)

THE LARGE INTESTINE MERIDIAN (LI)

Energy disturbance in the large intestine meridian affecting physical and physiological levels can give rise to the following symptoms:

Abdominal pain
Acne on the face, sides of
 the mouth and nose
Asthma after 5 a.m.
Arthritis of the shoulder
 joint
Arthritis of the knee joint
Arthritis of the index
 finger
Arthritis of the wrist joint
Arthritis of the lateral part
 of the elbow and hip
Bad breath
Blisters in the lower gum
Bursitis
Dermatitis
Dry mouth and thirst
Eczema
Fatigue
Feeling better after a
 bowel movement
Feeling tired after a bowel
 movement
Flatulence
Inflammation of lower
 gum

Intestinal colic
Itching of the body
Loose stools or constipation
Lower backache
Headaches over the eyes
Muscle spasms and pain of
lateral aspect of thigh, knee
 and below knee.
Motor impairment of the
fingers
 Pain in the knee
Pain in the shoulder,
 shoulder blade and back of
 the neck
Pain and swelling of the
 index finger
Pain in the heel
Sciatic pain
Swollen cervical glands
Skin rashes
Skin tags
Sinusitis
Tenosynovitis
Tennis elbow
Toothache
Warts on the skin.

Say Good-bye to Headaches

Energy disturbance in the large intestine meridian affecting the cellular level can cause the following:

Guilt

Confusion

Brain fog

Bad dreams

 dwelling on past memory

Crying spells

Defensiveness

Inability to recall dreams

Nightmares

Nostalgia

Rolling restlessly in sleep

Seeking sympathy

Talking in the sleep and Weeping

Essential Nutrients to Strengthen the Large Intestine Meridian

Vitamins A, D, E, C, B, especially B_1, wheat, wheat bran, oat bran, yogurt, and roughage.

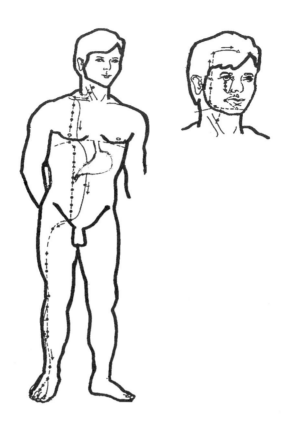

FIGURE 4-3

STOMACH MERIDIAN (ST)

THE STOMACH MERIDIAN (ST)

Energy disturbance in the stomach meridian affecting physical and physiological levels can give rise to the following symptoms:

Abdominal Pains & distention
Acid reflux disorders
Acne on the face and neck
ADD & ADHD
Anorexia
Autism
Bad breath
Black/ blue marks on the
  leg below the knee
Bipolar disorders
Blemishes
Bulimia
Chest muscle pain
Coated tongue
Coldness in the lower limbs
Cold sores in the mouth
Delirium
Depression
Dry nostrils
Dyslexia
Excessive hunger
Facial paralysis
Fever blisters
Fibromyalgia
Flushed face
Frontal headache
Herpes

Heat boils (painful acne) in
the upper front of the body
Headaches over the forehead
Hiatal hernia
High fever
Learning disability
Insomnia due to nervousness
Itching on the skin & rashes
Migraine headaches
Manic depressive disorders
Nasal polyps
Nausea
Nosebleed
Pain on the upper jaws
Pain in the mid-back
Pain in the eye
Seizures
Sensitivity to cold
Sore throat
Sores on the gums & tongue
Sweating
Swelling on the neck
Temporomandibular joint
  problem
Unable to relax the mind
Upper gum diseases
Vomiting

Energy disturbance in the stomach meridian affecting the cellular level can cause the following:

Disgust
Bitterness
Aggressive behaviors

Attention deficit disorders
Butterfly sensation in the
    stomach

Essential Nutrients to Strengthen the Stomach Meridian

B complex vitamins especially B_{12}, B_6, B_3 and folic acid.

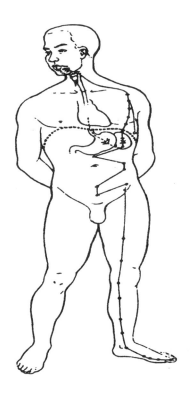

FIGURE 4-4

THE SPLEEN MERIDIAN (SP)

THE SPLEEN MERIDIAN (SP)

Energy disturbance in the spleen meridian affecting physical and physiological levels can give rise to the following symptoms:

Abnormal smell
Abnormal taste
Abnormal uterine bleeding
Absence of menstruation
Alzheimer's disease
Autism
Bitter taste in the mouth
Bleeding from the mucous
  membrane
Bleeding under the skin
Bruises under the skin
Carpal tunnel syndrome
Chronic gastroenteritis
Cold sores on the lips
Coldness of the legs
Cramps after the first day of
  menses
Depression
Diabetes
Dizzy spells
Dreams that make you tired
Emaciated muscles
Failing memory
Fatigue in general
Fatigue of the mind
Fatigued limbs
Feverishness
Fibromyalgia
Fingers and hands-numbness
Fluttering of the eyelids
Frequent
Generalized edema
Hard lumps in the abdomen
Hemophilia

Hemorrhoids
Hyperglycemia
Hypertension
Hypoglycemia
Inability to make decisions
Incontinence of urine or stool
Indigestion
Infertility
Insomnia: usually unable to fall
asleep
Intractable pain anywhere in the
body
Intuitive and prophetic behaviors
Irregular periods
Lack of enthusiasm
Lack of interest in anything
Lethargy
Light-headedness
Loose stools
Nausea
Obesity
Pain and stiffness of the fingers
Pain in the great toes
Pallor
Pedal edema
Pencil-like thin stools with
undigested food particles
Poor memory
Prolapse of the bladder
Prolapse of the uterus
Purpura
Reduced appetite
Sand-like feeling in the eyes
Scanty menstrual flow

Say Good-bye to Headaches

Sensation of heaviness in the
  body and head
 Sleep during the day
Slowing of the mind
Sluggishness
Schizophrenia
 Stiffness of the tongue
Sugar craving
 Swelling anywhere in the body
Swellings or pain with swelling
  of the toes and feet

Swollen eyelids
Swollen lips
Tingling or abnormal sensation
  in the tip of the fingers and
  palms
Varicose veins
Vomiting
Watery eyes

Energy disturbance in the spleen meridian affecting the cellular level can cause
the following:

Anxiety
Concern
Does not like crowds
Easily hurt
Gives more importance to self
Hopelessness
Irritable
Keeps feelings inside
Lack of confidence
Likes loneliness
Likes to be praised
Likes to take revenge

Lives through others
Low self esteem
Needs constant encouragement
Obsessive compulsive
  behavior
Over sympathetic to others
Unable to make decisions
Restrained
Shy/timid
Talks to self
Worry

Essential Nutrients to Strengthen the Spleen Meridian

Vitamin A, vitamin C, calcium, chromium, protein, berries, aspar-
agas, bioflavonoids, rutin, hesparin, hawthorn berries, oranges,
root vegetables, and sugar.

THE HEART MERIDIAN (HT)

Energy disturbance in the heart meridian affecting the Physical and pysiological level can cause the following:

Angina-like pains
Chest pains
Discomfort when reclining
Dizziness
Dry throat
Excessive perspiration
Feverishness
Headache
Heart palpitation
Insomnia—unable to fall asleep
When awakened in the middle
    of sleep

Heaviness in the chest
Hot palms and soles
Irritability
Mental disorders
Nervousness
Pain along the left arm
Pain along the scapula
Pain and fullness in the chest
Pain in the eye
Poor circulation
Shortness of breath
Shoulder pains

Energy disturbance in the heart meridian affecting the cellular level can cause the following:

Abusive nature
Aggression
Anger
Bad manners
Compassion and love
Compulsive behaviors
Does not like to make friends
Does not trust anyone
Easily upset
Excessive laughing or crying

Guilt
Hostility
Insecurity
Joy
Lack of emotions
overexcitement
Lack of love and compassion
Sadness
Self-confidence
Type A personality

Essential Nutrients to Strengthen the Heart Meridian

Calcium, vitamin C, vitamin E, fatty acids, selenium, potassium, sodium, iron, and B complex.

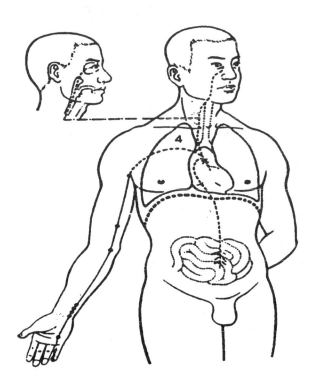

FIGURE 4-5

THE HEART MERIDIAN (HT)

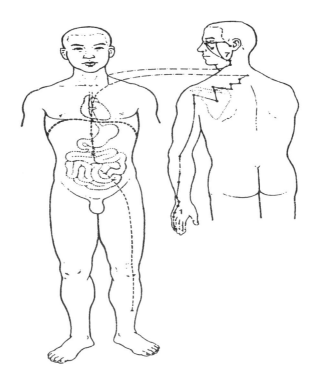

FIGURE 4-6

THE SMALL INTESTINE MERIDIAN (SI)

THE SMALL INTESTINE MERIDIAN (SI)

Energy disturbance in the small intestine meridian affecting physical and physiological levels can give rise to the following symptoms:

Abdominal fullness
Abdominal pain
Acne on the upper back
Bad breath
Bitter taste in the mouth
Constipation
Diarrhea
Distention of lower abdomen
Dry stool
Frozen shoulder
Knee pain
Night sweats

Numbness of the back of the
    shoulder and arm
Numbness of the mouth and
    tongue
Pain along the lateral aspect
    of the shoulder and arm
Pain in the neck
Pain radiating around the waist
Shoulder pain
Sore throat
Stiff neck

Energy disturbance in the small intestine meridian affecting the cellular level can cause the following:

Insecurity
Absentmindedness
Becoming too involved with
    details
Day dreaming
Easily annoyed
Emotional instability
Feeling of abandonment
Feeling shy
Having a tendency to be
    introverted and easily hurt
Irritability

Excessive joy or lack of
    joy
Lacking- confidence
Over excitement
Paranoia
Poor concentration
Sadness
Sighing
Sorrow
Suppressing deep
    sorrow

Essential Nutrients to Strengthen the Small Intestine Meridian

Vitamin B complex, vitamin D, vitamin E, acidophilus, yoghurt, fibers, fatty acids, wheat germ and whole grains.

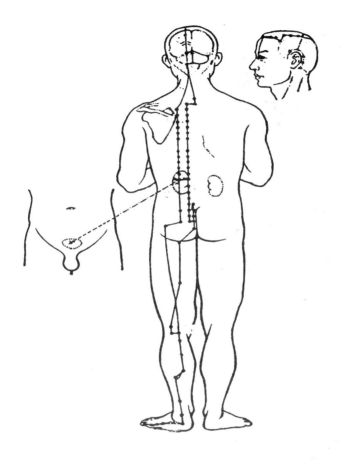

FIGURE 4-7
URINARY BLADDER MERIDIAN (UB)

URINARY BLADDER MERIDIAN (UB)

Energy disturbance in the Urinary Bladder meridian affecting physical and physiological levels can give rise to the following symptoms:

Arthritis of little finger & toe
Bloody urine
Burning or painful urination
Chills and fever
Disease of the eye
Frequent urination
Headaches at the back of the neck
Loss of bladder control
Lower backache and stiffness
lower abdominal discomfort
Mental disorders
Muscle wasting
Nasal congestion

Pain in the inner canthus
Pain and/or spasms along back
  of the leg, foot and lateral
    part of the sole & toes
Pain in the ankle (lateral part)
Pain along the meridian
Retention of urine
Sciatic neuralgia
Spasm behind the knee
Spasms of the calf muscles
Stiff neck
Weakness in the rectum and
  rectal muscle

Energy disturbance in the bladder meridian affecting the cellular level can cause the following:

Fright
Sadness
Disturbing and impure
  thoughts
Annoyed
Fearful
Unhappy

Frustrated
Highly irritable
Impatient
Inefficient
Insecure
Reluctant
Restless

Essential Nutrients to Strengthen the Bladder Meridian

Vitamin C, A, E, B complex, especially B_1, calcium, amino acids and trace minerals.

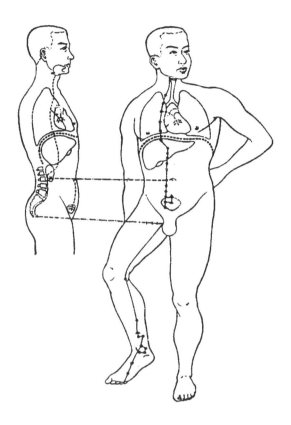

FIGURE   4-8

THE KIDNEY MERIDIAN   (KI)

THE KIDNEY MERIDIAN (KI)

Energy disturbance in the kidney meridian affecting physical and physiological levels can give rise to the following symptoms:

Bags under the eyes
Blurred vision
Burning or painful urination
Chronic diarrhea
Coldness in the back
Cold feet
Crave salt
Dark circles under the eyes
Dryness of the mouth
Excessive sleeping
Excessive salivation
Excessive thirst
Facial edema
Fatigue
Fever with chills
Frequent urination
Impotence
Irritability
Light- headedness
Lower backache

Motor impairment
Muscular atrophy of the foot
Nagging mild asthma
Nausea
Pain in the sole of the foot
Pain in the posterior aspect of the leg or thigh
Pain in the ears
Poor memory
Poor concentration
Poor appetite
Puffy eyes
Ringing in the ears
Sore throat
Spasms of the ankle and feet
Swelling in the legs
Swollen ankles and vertigo

Energy disturbance in the kidney meridian affecting the cellular level can cause the following:

Fear
Terror
Caution
Confused

Indecision
Paranoia
Seeks attention
Unable to express feelings

Essential Nutrients to Strengthen the Kidney Meridian

Vitamins A, E, B, essential fatty acids, amino acids, sodium chloride (table salt), trace minerals, calcium and iron.

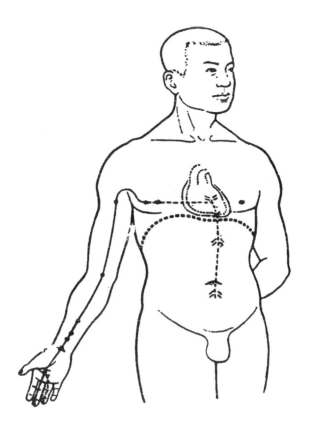

FIGURE 4-9

THE PERICARDIUM MERIDIAN (PC)

THE PERICARDIUM MERIDIAN (PC)

Energy disturbance in the pericardium meridian affecting physical and physiological levels can give rise to the following symptoms:

Chest pain
Contracture of the arm or elbow
Excessive appetite
Fainting spells
Flushed face
Frozen shoulder
Fullness in the chest
Heaviness in the chest
Hot palms and soles
Impaired speech
Irritability
Motor impairment of the tongue
Nausea

Nervousness
Pain in the anterior part of the thigh
Pain in the eyes
Pain in the medial part of the knee
Palpitation
Restricting movements
Sensation of hot or cold
Slurred speech
Spasms of the elbow and arm

Energy Disturbance in the Pericardium Meridian Affecting the Cellular Level Can Cause the Following:

Extreme joy
Fear of heights
Heaviness in the chest due to emotional overload
Heaviness in the head
Hurt
Imbalance in sexual energy like never having enough sex
In some cases no desire for sex

Jealousy
Light sleep with dreams
Manic disorders
Over- excitement
Regret
Sexual tension
Shock
Stubbornness
Various phobias

Essential Nutrients to Strengthen the Pericardium Meridian

Vitamin E, Vitamin C, Chromium, Manganese, Lotus seed, and Trace Minerals.

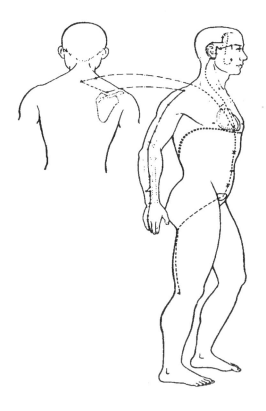

FIGURE 4-10

THE TRIPLE WARMER MERIDIAN (TW)

Say Good-bye to Headaches

THE TRIPLE WARMER MERIDIAN (TW)

Energy disturbance in the triple warmer meridian affecting physical and physiological levels can give rise to the following symptoms:

Abdominal pain
Always feels hungry even after eating a full meal
Constipation
Deafness
Distention
Dysuria
Edema
Enuresis
Excessive thirst
Excessive hunger
Fever in the late evening
Frequent urination
Indigestion
Hardness and fullness in the lower abdomen
Pain in the medial part of the knee
Pain in the shoulder and upper arm
Pain behind the ear
Pain in the cheek and jaw
Redness in the eye
Shoulder pain
Swelling and pain in the throat
Vertigo

Energy disturbance in the triple warmer meridian affecting the cellular level can cause the following:

Depression
Deprivation
Despair
Emptiness
Excessive Emotion
Grief
Hopelessness
Phobias

Essential nutrients to strengthen the triple warmer meridian

Iodine, trace minerals, vitamin C, calcium, fluoride, radish, onion, zinc, vanadium, and water.

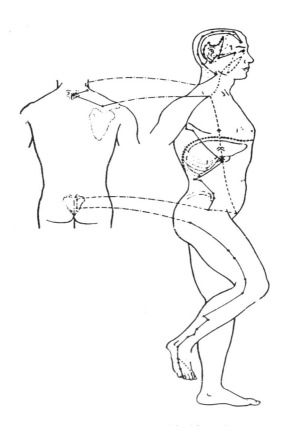

FIGURE   4-11

THE GALL BLADDER MERIDIAN (GB)

THE GALL BLADDER MERIDIAN (GB)

Energy disturbance in the gall bladder meridian affecting physical and physio-logical levels can give rise to the following symptoms:

A heavy sensation in the right
upper part of the abdomen
Abdominal bloating
Alternating fever and chills
Ashen complexion
Bitter taste in the mouth
Burping after meals
Chills
Deafness
Dizziness
Fever
Headaches on the sides of the
head
Heartburn after fatty foods
Hyperacidity
Moving arthritis
Pain in the jaw

Nausea with fried foods
Pain in the eye
Pain in the hip
Pain and cramps along the
anterolateral wall
Poor digestion of fats
Sciatic neuralgia
Sighing
Stroke-like condition
Swelling in the submaxillary
region
Tremors
Twitching
Vision disturbances
Vomiting
Yellowish complexion

Energy Disturbance in the Gall Bladder Meridian Affecting the Cellular Level Can Cause the Following:

Aggression
Complaining all the time
Rage

Fearful, finding faults with
others
Unhappiness.

Essential Nutrients to Strengthen the Gall Bladder Meridian

Vitamin A, apples, lemon, calcium, linoleic acids and oleic acids (for example, pine nuts, olive oil).

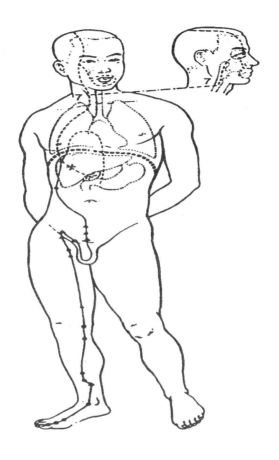

FIGURE 4-12

THE LIVER MERIDIAN (LIV)

THE LIVER MERIDIAN (LIV)

Energy disturbance in the liver meridian affecting physical and physiological levels can give rise to the following symptoms:

Abdominal pain
Blurred vision
Dark urine
Dizziness
Enuresis
Bright colored bleeding during
  menses
Feeling of obstruction in the
  throat
Fever
Hard lumps in the upper
  abdomen
Headache at the top of the head
Hernia
Hemiplegia
Irregular menses

Jaundice
Loose stools
Pain in the intercostal region
Pain in the breasts
Pain in the lower abdomen
Paraplegia
PMS
Reproductive organ
  disturbances
Retention of urine
Seizures
Spasms in the extremities
Stroke-like condition
Tinnitus
Vertigo
Vomiting.

Energy disturbance in the liver meridian affecting the cellular level can cause the following:

Anger
Irritability
Aggression
Assertion

Rage
Shouting
Talking loud
Type A personality

Essential Nutrients to Strengthen the Liver Meridian

Beets, green vegetables, vitamin A, trace minerals, vitamin F

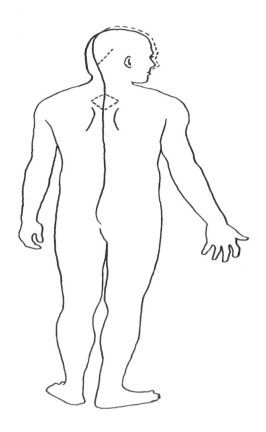

FIGURE 4-13

THE GOVERNING VESSEL MERIDIAN (GV)

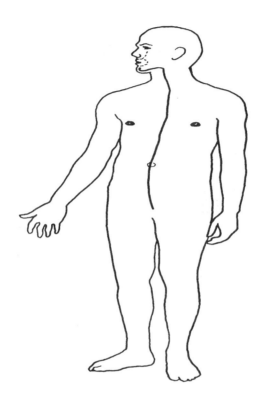

FIGURE 4-14

THE CONCEPTION VESSEL MERIDIAN (CV, REN)

THE GOVERNING VESSEL MERIDIAN (GV)

Energy disturbance in the governing vessel meridian affecting physical, physiological and psychological levels can give rise to various mixed symptoms of other yang meridians.

This channel supplies the brain and spinal region and intersects the liver channel at the vertex. Obstruction of its Chi may result in symptoms such as stiffness and pain along the spinal column. Deficient Chi in the channel may produce a heavy sensation in the head, vertigo and shaking. Energy blockages in this meridian (which passes through the brain) may be responsible for certain mental disorders. Febrile diseases are commonly associated with the governing vessel channel and because one branch of the channel ascends through the abdomen, when the channel is unbalanced, its Chi rushes upward toward the heart. Symptoms such as colic, constipation, enuresis, hemorrhoids and functional infertility may result.

THE CONCEPTION VESSEL MERIDIAN (CV, REN)

Energy disturbance in the conception vessel meridian affecting physical, physiological and psychological levels can give rise to various mixed symptoms of other yin meridians.

The conception vessel channel is the confluence of the Yin channels. Therefore, abnormality along the conception vessel channel will appear principally in pathological symptoms of the Yin channels, especially symptoms associated with the liver and kidneys. Its function is closely related with pregnancy and, therefore, has intimate links with the kidneys and uterus. If its Chi is deficient, infertility or other disorders of the urogenital system may result. Leukorrhea, irregular menstruation, colic, low libido, impotency, male and female infertility are associated with the conception vessel channel.

Any allergen can cause blockage in one or more meridians at the same time. If it is causing blockages in only one meridian, the patient may demonstrate symptoms related to that particular meridian. The intensity of the symptoms will depend on the severity of the blockage. The patient may suffer from one symptom, many symptoms or all the symptoms of this blocked meridian.

Sometimes a patient can have many meridians blocked at the same time. In such cases, the patient may demonstrate a variety of symptoms, one symptom from each meridian or many symptoms from certain meridians and one or two from other. Some patients with blockage in one meridian can demonstrate just one symptom from the list, but it may be with great intensity.

Some individuals, even though they have energy disturbances in multiple meridians, may not show any symptoms. Such patients might have a better immune system than others. Variations with all these possibilities can make diagnosis difficult in some cases.

CHAPTER 5

NAET® TESTING PROCEDURES

W hen a person comes close to the energy field of a substance, if that energy field happens to be incompatible to the individual, then a repulsion of the two energy fields take place. The substance that is capable of producing the repulsion between the energy fields of the individual and the substance itself is considered an allergen to the particular individual. We frequently go near allergens and interact with their energies without recognizing this repulsive action, whether from foods, drinks, chemicals, environmental substances, animals or other humans. This causes energy disturbances in the meridians; thereby causing imbalances in the body. The imbalances cause illnesses, which create disorganization in body functions. The disorganization of the body and its functions involve the vital organs, their associated muscle groups, and nerve roots which can give rise to brain disorders. To prevent the allergen from causing further disarray after producing the initial blockage, the brain sends messages to every cell of the body to reject the presence of the allergen. This rejection will appear as repulsion, and the repulsion will produce different symptoms related to the affected organs.

Our body has an amazing way of telling us when we are in trouble. If we went for help at the earliest hint of need, we would save ourselves from unnecessary pain and agony. As a matter of habit, we often have to be hurting severely before we seek help. This applies to chemical allergies, too. If we have a way to identify the allergens that can possibly cause reactions on our body way before we get exposed to them, we can simply avoid them and won't have to suffer the the consequences. Now we have a way to do just that through NAET® testing procedures (NAET® Testing procedures are described in the following pages).

When we go near allergens, we may receive various clues from the brain if we are very aware of our own body sensitivities. Some of the examples of such body awareness are: itching, sneezing, coughing spells, stretching the body, yawning, feeling of fatigueness, pain anywhere in the body, etc. can happen when we come near an allergen. We can demonstrate these changes by testing the strength of any part of the body in the presence and absence of the allergen. A strong muscle of the arm, hand or leg can be used for this test. Test a strong muscle for its strength away from the allergen, and then test it again in the presence of the allergen and compare the strength. The muscle will stay strong without any allergen near the body, but will weaken in the presence of an allergen. This response of the muscle can be used to our advantage to demonstrate the presence of an allergen near us.

NEUROMUSCULAR SENSITIVITY TESTING
(NST-NAET ®)

NST is one of the tools used by NAET® specialists to test imbalances and allergies in the body. The same muscle response testing can also be used to detect various allergens that cause imbalances in the body.

Neuromuscular sensitivity testing can be performed in the following ways (Illustrations of different types of NST can be seen on the following pages).

1. Standard NST can be done in standing, sitting or lying positions.

2. The "Oval Ring Test" can be used in testing yourself, and on a very strong person with a strong arm.

3. Surrogate testing can be used to test an infant, invalid person, extremely strong or very weak person, or an animal. The surrogate's muscle is tested by the tester, and the subject maintains skin-to-skin contact with the surrogate while being tested. The surrogate does not get affected by the testing. NAET® treatments can also be administered through the surrogate very effectively without causing any interference with the surrogate's energy.

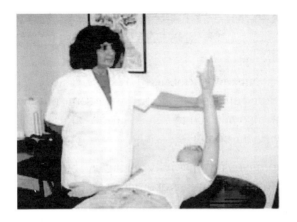

FIGURE 1
NST WITHOUT ALLERGEN

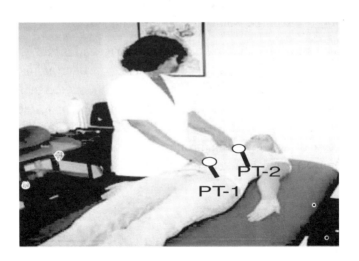

FIGURE 2
INITIAL BALANCING

NST PROCEDURE

Two people are required to perform standard neuromuscular sensitivity testing: the tester, and the subject. The subject can be tested lying down, standing, or sitting. The lying-down position is the most convenient for both tester and subject; it also achieves more accurate results.

Step 1:   The subject lies on a firm surface with the left arm raised 45-90 degrees to the body with the palm facing outward and the thumb pointing toward the big toe.

Step 2: The tester stands on the subject's (right) side. The subject's right arm is kept to his/her side with the palm either kept open to the air, or in a loose fist. The fingers should not touch any material, fabric or any part of the table the arm is resting on because this can give wrong test results. The tester's left palm is contacting the subject's left wrist (Figure 5-1).

Step 3: It is essential to test a strong predetermined muscle (PDM) to get accurate results. The tester using the left arm tries to push the raised arm toward the subject's left big toe. The subject resists the push. The arm, or pre-determined indicator muscle, remains strong if the subject is well balanced at the time of testing. If the muscle or raised arm is weak and gives way under pressure without the presence of an allergen, either the subject is not balanced, or the tester is performing the test improperly; for example, the tester might be trying to overpower the subject. The subject does not need to gather up strength from other muscles in the body to resist the tester. Only 5 to 10 pounds of pressure needs to be applied for three to five seconds. If the muscle shows weakness, the tester will be able to judge the difference with only that small amount of pressure.

Step 4: This step is used if the patient is found to be out of balance as indicated by the PDM presenting weak without the presence of an allergen. The tester then uses the balancing points by placing the fingertips of right hand at Point 1. The left hand is placed on Point 2 (see below and figure 5-2). The tester massages these two points gently clockwise with the fingertips about 20-30 seconds, and then repeats steps 2 and 3. If the PDM tests strong, continue on to step 5.

MORE ON STEP-4

Point 1:

Name of the point: Sea of Energy

Location: Two finger-breadths below the navel, on the midline. According to Oriental medical theory, this is where the energy of the body is stored in abundance. When the body senses any danger around its energy field or when the body experiences energy disturbances, the energy supply is cut short and stored here. If you massage clockwise on that energy reservoir point, the energy will come out of this storage and travel to the part of the body where it is needed.

Point 2:

Name of the point: Dominating Energy

Location: In the center of the chest on the midline of the body, level with the fourth intercostal space. This is the energy dispenser department. According to Oriental medical theory, when the energy rises from the Sea of Energy, it goes straight to the Dominating Energy point. This is the point that controls and regulates the energy circulation or Chi flow in the body. From this point, the energy is distributed to different meridians, organs, tissues and cells as needed to help remove the energy disturbances in those affected areas. This is done by forcing energy circulation to flow from the energy distribution area (Point-2 on figure-2) to the affected meridian, then to the affected tissue in the meridian moving the energy into general circulation or we can say "move the energy from inside out". Continue this procedure for 30 seconds to one minute and repeat the NST. If the NST is found weak repeat the procedure until it gets strong. Check NST every 30 seconds. In a very sick individual it may be necessary to repeat this procedure for three or four times before the PDM becomes strong.

Step 5: If the PDM remains strong when tested - a sign that the subject is balanced - then the tester should put the suspected allergen into the palm of the subject's resting hand. When the subject's fingertips touch the allergen, the sensory receptors sense the allergen's charges and relay the message to the brain. If it is an incompatible charge, the strong PDM will go weak. If the charges are compatible to the body, the indicator muscle will remain strong. This way, you can test any number of items to determine the compatible and incompatible charges.

Much practice is needed to test and sense the differences properly. If you can't test properly or effectively the first few times, don't get discouraged. Practice makes one perfect.

NST is one of the most reliable methods of allergy tests, and it is fairly easy to learn and practice in every day life. The tester will develop confidence after getting enough practice. It also cuts out expensive laboratory work.

After considerable practice, some people are able to test very efficiently using these methods. It is very important for the

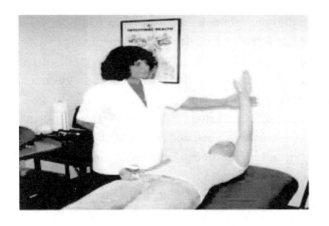

FIGURE   3
NST WITH ALLERGEN

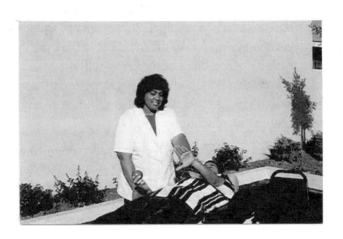

FIGURE   4
NST WEAK WITH ALLERGEN

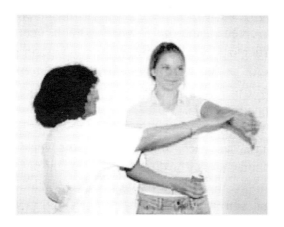

FIGURE 5
NST STANDING

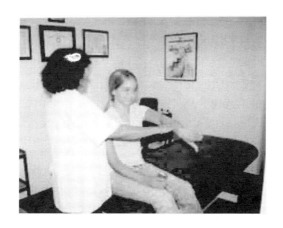

FIGURE 6
NST SITTING

chemically sensitive people to learn this simple testing technique to screen out the allergies before he/she gets exposed to them in order to prevent unexpected allergic reactions. After receiving NAET® Basic treatments from a trained NAET® practitioner, you can begin to test and screen your daily encountering allergens before using them. Then the offending substances can easily be avoided, or if it is unavoidable, be treated. Hundreds of new allergens are thrown into the world daily by chemical manufacturers who do not understand the predicament of allergic people. If you want to live in this world looking and feeling normal, you have to learn self-testing. It is not practical for anyone to treat thousands of allergens from their surroundings or go to an NAET® practitioner every day for the rest of one's life. If you learn to detect the allergies on your own, after treating for NAET® basics you can easily avoid most other allergens by testing prior to exposures.

"OVAL RING TEST" OR "O RING TEST"

The "Oval Ring Test" or "O Ring Test" can be used in self-testing (See figure 5-9). This can also be used to test a subject, if the subject is very strong physically with a strong arm and the tester is a physically weak person.

Step 1: The tester makes an "O" shape by opposing the little finger and thumb on the same hand (finger pad to finger pad). Then, with the index finger of the other hand he/she tries to separate the "O" ring against pressure. If the ring separates easily, the tester needs to be balanced as described above.

Step 2: If the "O" ring remains inseparable and strong, hold an allergen in the other hand, by the fingertips, and perform step 1 again. If the "O" ring separates easily, the person is allergic to the

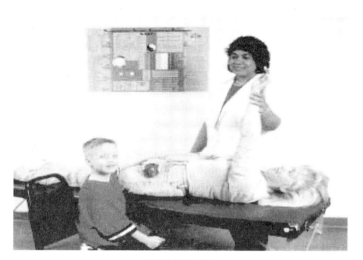

FIGURE 7
TESTING A TODDLER THROUGH A SURROGATE

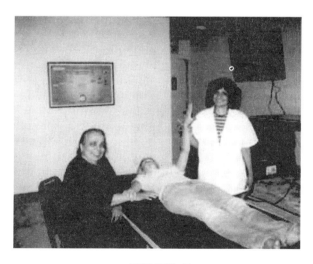

FIGURE 8
TESTING THROUGH A SURROGATE

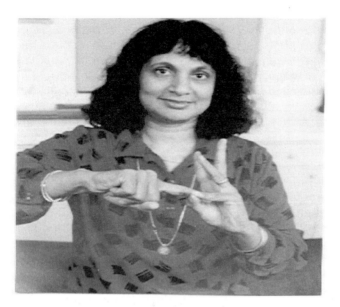

FIGURE 9
"O" RING TESTING

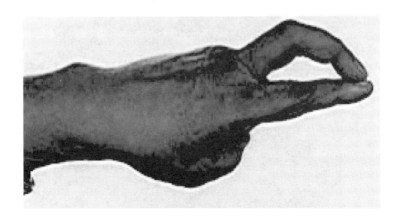

FIGURE 10
FINGER ON FINGER TESTING

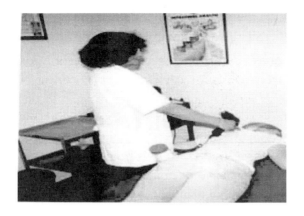

FIGURE 11
NAET TREATMENT

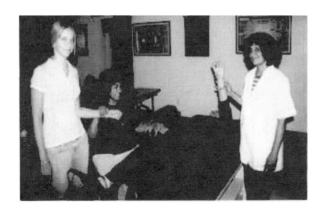

FIGURE 12
EXTENDED SURROGATE TESTING

substance in the hand. If the "O" ring remains strong, the substance is not an allergen.

After considerable practice, some people are able to test very efficiently using these methods. It is very important for allergic people to learn some form of self-testing technique to screen out contact with possible allergens to prevent allergic reactions in order to have freedom to live in this chemically polluted world. After receiving the basic 30-40 treatments from a NAET® practitioner, a person can test and avoid unexpected allergens. Hundreds of new allergens are thrown into the world daily by people who do not understand the predicament of allergic people. If you want to live in this world looking and feeling normal among normal people, you need to learn how to test on your own. It is not practical for people to treat thousands of allergens from their surroundings or go to a NAET® practitioner every day. If you learn to detect your allergies on your own after treating for NAET® basics, you can live without many health problems.

A TIP TO MASTER SELF-TESTING

Find two items, one that you are allergic to and another that you are not, for example an apple and a banana.

You are allergic to the apple and not allergic to the banana. Hold the apple in the right hand and do the "Oval Ring Test" as shown in the figure 5-7. The ring easily breaks. The first few times if it didn't break, make it happen intentionally. Now hold the banana and do the same test. This time the ring doesn't break. Put the banana down; rub your hands together for 30 seconds. Take the apple and repeat the testing. Practice this until you can sense the difference. When you can feel the difference between these two items you can test anything around you.

SURROGATE TESTING

This method can be very useful to test and determine the allergies of an infant, a child, a hyperactive child, an autistic child, disabled person, an unconscious person, an extremely strong, and a very weak person. You can also use this method to test an animal, plant, and a tree.

TESTING THROUGH AN EXTENDED SURROGATE

Extended surrogate testing is used when the patient is uncooperative, i.e. hyperactive, autistic, or frightened. Three people are needed for this test as shown in Figure 5-12. NAET® treatments can be administered through the extended surrogate very effectively without causing any interference to the surrogate's energy.

The surrogate's muscle is tested by the tester. It is very important to remember to maintain skin-to-skin contact between the surrogate and the subject during the procedure. If you do not, then the surrogate will receive the results of testing and treatment.

The testing or treatment does not affect the surrogate as long as the subject maintains uninterrupted skin-to-skin contact with the surrogate.

NST can be used to test any substance for allergies. Even human beings can be tested for each other in this manner. When allergic to another human (father, mother, son, daughter, grandfather, grandmother, spouse, caretaker, baby sitter, etc.) you or your child could experience similar symptoms just as you would with foods, chemicals, or materials.

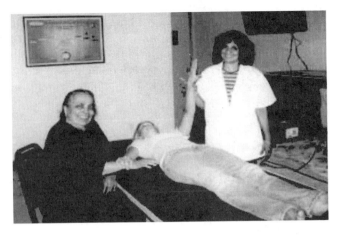

FIGURE 13
PERSON TO PERSON TESTING (A TO B)

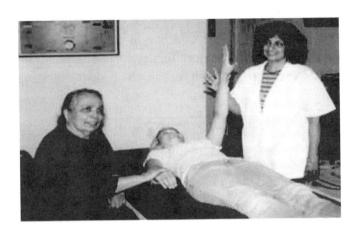

FIGURE 14
PERSON TO PERSON TESTING (B TO A)

ABOUT PERSON-TO-PERSON ALLERGIES

If people are allergic to each other, the allergy can affect a person in various ways: If the father and/or mother is allergic to the child, or child allergic to a parent or parents, the child can get sick or remain sick indefinitely. The same things can happen to the parents. If the husband is allergic to the wife or wife towards the husband, they might fight all the time and/or their health can be affected. The same things can happen among other family members. It is important to test family members and other immediate associates with your child for possible allergy, and if found, they should be treated for each other.

TESTING PERSON-TO-PERSON ALLERGIES

The subject lies down and touches the other person he or she wants tested (Figures 5-13 and 5-14). The tester pushes the arm of the subject in steps 2 and 3 above. If the subject is allergic to the second person, the indicator muscle goes weak. If the subject is not allergic, the indicator muscle remains strong. This is done through a surrogate in autistic children. Sometimes, one needs to test an autistic or hyperactive child through an extended surrogate because the child may be violent or too strong for one surrogate to handle.

Using the methods described in this chapter, the tester can screen each and every food, drink, vitamins, medications, fabrics, chemicals, etc. before the headache person exposes herself or himself to the substance. If you find them as allergens, test more items until you can find some non-allergic products to use in your daily life. Of course, you have the option to treat for them and make non-allergic or avoid them and never use them again.

<u>Say Goodbye to Headaches</u>

If we can teach these simple testing skills to all headache victims and their families, guardians, caretakers, and their doctors, as well as encourage them to use non-allergic products or NAET® treated products in their daily use, individuals can eliminate or reduce headaches and can also lead a healthy and happy life.

NST is a variation of MRT (muscle response testing). It is an important tool used by kinesiologists. Practiced in this country since 1964, it was originated by Dr. George Goodheart and his associates. The late Dr. John F. Thie advocated this method through the "Touch for Health" Foundation in Malibu, California. For more information and books available on the subject, interested readers can write to "Touch For Health" Foundation.

CHAPTER 6

NAET® Home-Help

Many people take vitamins, enzymes and mineral supplements nowadays. The quality of the food is far worse than years ago. The food products we buy in the market have less food value than necessary, so it has become a necessity to supplement our food if we are to prevent malnutrition.

Vitamins and trace minerals are essential to life. Vitamins are compounds required for biochemical reactions, which cannot be synthesized in higher animals but must be obtained in diet. Vitamins are generally classified in two categories. Water soluble (B vitamins, folate, biotin, pantothenate) are stored very little and have to be supplied frequently. Fat soluble vitamins (vitamin A, D, E, K) can be stored in tissue and thus pose a risk for toxicity when taken in excess. Vitamins are precursors of cofactors in numerous chemical reactions in the body. Examples of some functions are:

B vitamins are used in enzymatic functions, nerve functions thus maintaining a sound mental health, sleep functions, immune functions and reduce everyday stress.

Vitamin A is involved in the visual processes and regulation of transcription as well as to improve and maintain immune functions.

Vitamin C and E are natural antioxidants and helps to reduce free radicals and internal toxins thus in reducing allergic reactions.

Vitamin K is necessary in the coagulation of blood, etc.

Vitamin D is important in bone formation and for absorption of calcium in the body. It is formed by the body when the skin is exposed to sunlight (ultraviolet light).

Vitamins and trace minerals are micronutrients, and the body needs them in small amounts. The lack of these essential elements even though they are needed in minute amounts can create various impairments and tissue damage in the body.

Water, carbohydrates, fats, proteins and bulk minerals like calcium, magnesium, sodium, potassium and phosphorus are considered to be macronutrients, taken into the body via regular food. They are needed in larger amounts. Both macro- and micronutrients are not only necessary to produce energy for our daily bodily functions, but also for growth and development of the body and mind.

Using macronutrients (food & drinks) and micronutrients (vitamins and trace minerals), the body creates some essential chemicals, enzymes and hormones. These are the foundations of human bodily functions. Enzymes are the catalysts or simple activators in the chemical reactions that are continually taking place in the body. Without the appropriate vitamins and trace minerals, the production and functions of the enzymes will be incomplete. Prolonged deficiency of these vitamins and minerals can produce immature or incomplete enzyme production, protein synthesis, cell mutation, immature RNA, DNA synthesis, etc., which can mimic various organic diseases in the body. The effect of the deficiency will cause the weakest tissue to suffer most. In patients with headaches, head is the weak area in their bodies and deficiency of nutrients can trigger headaches in them.

Deficiency of vitamins, minerals and enzymes can cause headaches in some people. Deficiency of vitamins and other essential nutrients in the body can be due to poor intake and absorption.

Poor absorption can be due to allergies and sensitivities to the nutrients or nutritional elements. This is the reason NAET® Basic allergens desensitization treatments stress treating essential nutrients first.

Fat-soluble vitamins are stored for longer periods of time in the body's fatty tissues and the liver. When you are allergic to fat soluble vitamins, you begin to store them in unwanted places of the body. Some of the abnormal fat-soluble vitamin storage can be seen as lipomas, warts, skin tags, benign tumors inside or outside the body, etc.

Taking vitamins and minerals in their proper balance is important for the correct functioning of all vitamins. Excess consumption of an isolated vitamin or mineral can produce unpleasant symptoms of that particular nutrient. High doses of one element can also cause depletion of other nutrients in the body, leading to other problems. Most of these vitamins work synergistically, complementing and/or strengthening each other's function.

Vitamins and minerals should be taken with meals unless specified otherwise. Oil-soluble vitamins should be taken before meals, and water-soluble vitamins should be taken between or after meals. But when you are taking megadoses of any of these, they should always be taken with or after meals. Vitamins and minerals, as nutritional supplements taken with meals, will supply the missing nutrients in our daily diets.

Synthetic vitamins are produced in a laboratory from isolated chemicals with similar characteristics to natural vitamins. Although there are no major chemical differences between a vitamin found in food and one created in a laboratory, natural supplements do not contain other unnatural ingredients. Supplements that are not labeled natural may include coal tars, artificial coloring, preservatives, sugars, and starches, as well as other binding agents and additives. Vitamins labeled natural may not contain vitamins that have not been extracted from a natural food source. One must select carefully. Some binding substances are necessary to prepare vitamins in tablets or capsule form. Capsules take less amount of additives. You should use a product with minimum number of binding products. Vegetarian capsules are available in the market even though the cost is slightly high.

VITAMIN A

Clinical studies have proven vitamin A and beta-carotene to be very powerful immune-stimulants and protective agents.

Vitamin A is necessary for proper vision and in preventing night blindness, skin disorders, and acne. It protects the body against colds, influenza and other infections. It enhances immunity, helps heal ulcers and wounds and maintains the epithelial cell tissue. It is necessary for the growth of bones and teeth.

Vitamin A works best with B complex, vitamin D, vitamin E, calcium, phosphorus and zinc. Zinc is needed to get vitamin A out of the liver, where it is usually stored. Large doses of vitamin A should be taken only under proper supervision, because it can accumulate in the body and become toxic.

VITAMIN D

Vitamin D is often called the sunshine vitamin. It is a fat-soluble vitamin, acquired through sunlight or food sources. Vitamin D is absorbed from foods, through the intestinal wall, after they are ingested. Smog reduces the vitamin D producing rays of the sun. Dark-skinned people and sun-tanned people do not absorb vitamin D from the sun. Vitamin D helps the utilization of calcium and phosphorus in the human body. When there is an allergy to vitamin D, the vitamin is not absorbed into the body through foods, or from the sun. People with an allergy to vitamin D can exhibit deficiency syndromes: rickets, severe tooth decay, softening of teeth and bones, osteomalacia, osteoporosis, sores on the skin, blisters on the skin while walking in the sun, severe sunburns when exposed to the sun, etc. Sometimes allergic persons can show toxic symptoms if they take vitamin D without clearing its allergy. These symptoms include mental confusion, headaches, unusual thirst, sore eyes, itching skin, vomiting, diarrhea, urinary urgency, calcium deposits in the blood vessels and bones, restlessness in the sun, inability to bear heat, sun radiation, electrical radiation, emotional imbalance like depression, suicidal thoughts in the winter when the sunlight is diminished. Some people in Alaska and other cold countries suffer emotional instabilities during winter (Seasonal affective Disorders or SAD) where they have a few hours of daylight in winter. When they get treated for vitamin D, and combinations, with NAET, they do not suffer from depression anymore. From this experience, it should be assumed that vitamin D is very necessary to maintain mental stability. Vitamin D works best with vitamin A, vitamin C, choline, calcium, and phosphorus.

VITAMIN E

Vitamin E is an antioxidant. The body needs zinc in order to maintain the proper levels of vitamin E in the blood. Vitamin E is a fat-soluble vitamin and is stored in the liver, fatty tissues, heart, muscles, testes, uterus, blood, adrenal and pituitary glands. Vitamin E is excreted in the feces if too much is taken.

VITAMIN K

Vitamin K is needed for blood clotting and bone formation. Vitamin K is necessary to convert glucose into glycogen for storage in the liver. Vitamin K is a fat-soluble vitamin, very essential to the formation of prothrombin, a blood-clotting material. It helps in the blood-clotting mechanism, prevents hemorrhages (nosebleeds and intestinal bleeding) and helps reduce excessive menstrual flow.

An allergy to vitamin K can produce deficiency syndromes such as prolonged bleeding time, intestinal diseases like sprue, etc., and colitis.

VITAMIN B

Approximately 15 vitamins make up the B complex family. Each one of them has unique, very important functions in the body. If the body does not absorb and utilize any or all of the B-vitamins, various health problems can result. B complex vitamins are very essential for emotional, physical and physiological well being of the human body. It is a nerve food, so it is necessary for the proper growth and maintenance of the nervous system and brain function. It also keeps the nerves well fed so that nerves are kept calm and the autistic person can maintain a good mental attitude.

B-vitamins are seen in almost all foods we eat. Cooking and heating destroy some of them, others are not destroyed by processing or preparation. People who are allergic to B-vitamins can get mild to severe reactions just by eating the foods alone. If they are supplemented with vitamin B complex, without being aware of the allergies, such people can get exaggerated reactions. One has to be very cautious when taking B complex, commonly called stress vitamins.

Dr. Carlton Frederic, in his book, "Psychonutrition," tried to point out that nutritional deficiencies are the causes of most of the mental irritations such as extreme anger, severe mood swings, bipolar diseases, schizophrenic disorders, frontal lobe disorders, anxiety disorders, attention deficit disorders, hyperactivity disorders, various neurological disorders, mental sicknesses including mild to moderate to severe psychiatric disorders. He tried to prove his theory by giving large doses of vitamin B complex, especially B-12, to some of the psychiatric patients. Fifty percent of the patients got better, were cured of their mental sickness and went back to live normal lives. But another 50 percent made no progress or got worse. He couldn't explain why the other 50% got worse. His theory was ridiculed and his treatment protocol with mega B complex vitamin therapy for mental disorders was thrown out for want of proof. He did not think in the direction of allergies. When I discovered the allergic connection, I tried to contact him to let him know that his theory was absolutely right and I had proof to support his theory. Unfortunately, I was a year late to reach him. He had passed away a year before my discovery of NAET.

A few minerals are extremely essential for our daily functions. While some metals and trace minerals are mentioned here, for more information on other minerals, please refer to the appropriate references in the bibliography.

CALCIUM

Calcium is one of the essential minerals in the body. Calcium works with phosphorus, magnesium, iron, vitamins A, C and D. Calcium helps to maintain strong bones and healthy teeth. It regulates the heart functions and helps to relax the nerves and muscles. It induces relaxation and sleep.

Deficiencies in calcium can result in rickets, osteomalacia, osteoporosis, hyperactivity, restlessness, inability to relax, generalized aches and pains, joint pains, formation of bone spurs, backaches, PMS, cramps in the legs and heavy menstrual flow.

IRON

Poor diet is certainly one cause of iron deficiency but if you are allergic to iron, you do not absorb iron. Iron is absorbed better in the acid medium (stomach) but in the intestine where the digestive juices are basic, iron does not absorb well. If you have a deficiency of iron, or if you have an allergy to iron and base in combination, all iron containing food can cause bloating and abdominal distention. Iron deficiency results in anemia. If you are allergic to iron, and if you supplement with iron or eat iron-containing foods, you may experience various allergic reactions like dry mouth, fatigue, dizziness, nausea, loss of appetite, restlessness, a short attention span, feeling extreme cold, cold limbs, internal cold and tremors, cold extremities, feels better in warm weather, poor circulation in the fingers and toes, varicose veins and fragile arteries, hair loss, insomnia, swelling of the feet and ankles, etc. Iron deficiency also can give rise to above symptoms. Iron is also necessary to maintain the health of blood cells especially red blood cells. This improves the absorption of oxygen and elimination of carbon dioxide and other toxins from blood. Iron plays an important role in awareness and alertness. An imbalance of iron in the blood causes sluggish synaptic functions in the nerve endings causing the neurotransmitters to function poorly resulting in behavior and learning disability in young children. So good assimilation and utilization of iron is necessary for body's natural detoxification and maintenance function. Vitamin C can enhance the iron absorption. A high fiber diet, and the repeated daily use of laxatives can deplete iron from your body. Drinking tea can deplete iron in the body. Drinking tea (tannic acid) with meals can inhibit the iron absorption from food.

Food sources: chicken liver, beef liver, beef, crab, soybean, blackstrap molasses, spinach, beets, beet green, beef, potato, scallops, sunflower seeds, pistachio, broccoli, cashew nuts, lima beans, Swiss chard, turkey dark-meat, lobster, tuna, almonds, sesame seeds, peanuts, peas, prunes, apricot, Brussels sprouts, cod, raisins, haddock, and endive.

CHROMIUM

Chromium is a natural insulin regulator. It is essential for insulin to work efficiently in our bodies. Insulin is required to remove glucose (sugar) from the blood. Chromium helps the insulin to do its job so that blood sugar can be kept at a normal range.

Food sources: sugar, whole grains, wheat germ, corn, corn oil, brewers yeast, mushrooms, red meat, liver, shellfish, clams and chicken.

COBALT

Cobalt is essential to form quality red blood cells, since it is part of vitamin B-12. Deficiency results in B-12 anemia. Multiple chemically sensitive people have low tolerance to any external smells like gasoline, smoke, chemical fumes, sprays, perfumes, etc. Maintaining a good level of cobalt along with selenium and molybdenum helps to reduce the smell-sensitivity in MCS people. If they are allergic to any of the trio, they should be treated singly or in combination before supplementation.

Food sources: green leafy vegetables, milk, buckwheat, figs, red meat, liver, kidney, oyster, and clams.

COPPER

Copper is required to convert the body's iron into hemoglobin. Combined with the thyroxin, it helps to produce the pigment factor for hair and skin. It is essential for utilization of vitamin C. Deficiency results in anemia and edema. Toxicity symptoms and allergic symptoms are insomnia, hair loss, irregular menses, joint pains, arthritis, headaches and depression.

Food sources: almonds, green beans, peas, green leafy vegetables, whole wheat, other whole grains, dried beans, prunes, raisins, beef-liver, shellfish, and fish.

FLUORIDE

Sodium fluoride is often added to drinking water. Calcium fluoride is seen in natural food sources. Fluorine decreases chances of dental carries, (too much can discolor teeth). It also strengthens the bones. Deficiency leads to tooth decay. Toxicity and allergy symptoms include dizziness, nausea, vomiting, fatigue, poor appetite, skin rashes, itching, yeast infections, mental confusion, muscle spasms, mental fogginess and arthritis. Treatment for fluoride will eliminate possible allergies.

Food sources: fluoridated water, gelatin, sunflower seeds, milk, cheese, carrots, almonds, green leafy vegetables and fish.

IODINE

Two thirds of the body's iodine is in the body's thyroid gland. Since the thyroid gland controls metabolism, and iodine influences the thyroid, an under supply of this mineral can result in weight gain, general fatigue and slow mental reaction. Iodine helps to keep the body thin, promotes growth, gives more energy, improves mental alertness, and promotes the growth of hair, nails and teeth. A deficiency in iodine can cause overweight, hypothyroidism, goiter and lack of energy.

Food sources: kelp, seafood, iodized salt, vegetables grown in iodine-rich soil, and onion.

MAGNESIUM

This is one of the important minerals to help with mental irritability, hyperactivity and headaches. Magnesium is necessary for the metabolism of calcium, vitamin C, phosphorus, sodium, potassium and vitamin A. It is essential for the normal functioning of nerves and muscles. People with headaches need more magnesium in their diet to maintain the stability of the nervous system. It also helps convert blood sugar into energy. It works as a natural tranquilizer, laxative and diuretic. Diuretics deplete magnesium.

Alcoholics, asthmatics and immune deficient people are deficient in magnesium.

Food sources: Nuts, soybean, green leafy vegetables, almonds, brown rice, whole grains, sesame seeds and sunflower seeds.

MANGANESE

Manganese helps to activate digestive enzymes in the body. It is important in the formation of thyroxin, the principal hormone of the thyroid gland. It is necessary for the proper digestion and utilization of food. Manganese is important in reproduction and the normal functioning of the central nervous system. It helps to eliminate fatigue, improves memory, reduces nervous irritability and relaxes the mind. A deficiency may result in recurrent attacks of dizziness and poor memory.

Food sources: green leafy vegetables, beets, blueberries, oranges, grapefruit, apricot, the outer coating of nuts, and grains, peas, kelp, raw egg yolk, nuts and wheat germ.

MOLYBDENUM

Molybdenum helps in carbohydrate and fat metabolism. It is a vital part of the enzyme responsible for iron utilization. It also helps reduce allergic reaction to smell in people.

Food sources: whole grains, brown rice, brewers yeast, legumes, buckwheat, millet, and dark green leafy vegetables.

PHOSPHORUS

Phosphorus is involved in all physiological chemical reactions in the body. It is necessary for normal bone and teeth formation, heart regularity, normal kidney function and proper fat and carbohydrate metabolism. It promotes growth, and it is essential for healthy gums and teeth. Vitamin D and calcium are essential for its proper functioning.

Food sources: whole grains, seeds, nuts, legumes, egg yolk, fish, corn, dried fruits, milk, cheese, yogurt, chicken, turkey and red meat.

POTASSIUM

Potassium works with sodium to regulate the body's water balance and to regulate the heart rhythm. It helps in clear thinking by sending oxygen to the brain. A deficiency in potassium results in edema, hypoglycemia, nervous irritability, and muscle weakness.

Food sources: vegetables, orange, banana, cantaloupe, tomatoes, mint leaves, water cress, potatoes, whole grains, seeds, nuts and cream of tartar.

SELENIUM

Selenium is an antioxidant. It works with vitamin E, slowing down the aging process. It prevents hardening of tissues and helps to retain youthful appearance. Selenium is also known to alleviate hot flashes and menopausal distress. It prevents dandruff. Some researchers have found selenium to neutralize certain carcinogens and provide protection from some cancers. It has been also found to reduce the sensitivity to smells and odors from plastics, formaldehyde, perfume, molds, smoke, and gasoline etc. It works when combined with cobalt and molybdenum.

Food sources: brewers yeast, wheat germ, kelp, sea water, sea salt, garlic, mushrooms, seafood, milk, eggs, whole grains, beef, dried beans, bran, onions, tomato and broccoli.

SODIUM

Sodium is essential for normal growth and normal body functioning. It works with potassium to maintain the sodium-potassium pump in the body. Potassium is found inside the cells and sodium is found outside.

Food sources: kelp, celery, romaine lettuce, watermelon, seafood, processed foods with salt, fast foods, table salt, fish, shellfish, carrots, beets, artichoke, dried beef, cured meats, bacon, ham, brain, kidney, watercress, sea weed, oats, avocado, Swiss chard, tomatoes, cabbage, cucumber, asparagus, pineapple, tap water, canned or frozen foods.

SULFUR

Sulfur is essential for healthy hair, skin and nails. It helps maintain the oxygen balance necessary for proper brain function. It works with B-complex vitamins for basic body metabolism. It is a part of tissue building amino acid. It tones up the skin and makes the hair lustrous and helps fight bacterial infection.

Food sources: radish, turnip, onion, celery, string beans, watercress, soybean, fish, meat, dried beans, eggs and cabbage.

VANADIUM

Vanadium prevents heart attacks. It inhibits the formation of cholesterol in blood vessels. It also regulates sugar metabolism.

Food sources: fish, seaweed, seafood.

ZINC

Zinc is essential to form certain enzymes and hormones in the body. It is very necessary for protein synthesis. It is important for blood stability and in maintaining the body's acid-alkaline balance. It is important in the development of reproductive organs and helps to normalize the prostate glands in males. It helps in treatment of mental disorders and speeds up healing of wounds and cuts on the body. Zinc helps with the growth of fingernails and eliminates cholesterol deposits in the blood vessels. It helps to improve the immune system.

Food sources: wheat bran, wheat germ, seeds, dried beans, peas, onions, mushrooms, brewers yeast, milk, eggs, oysters, herring, brown rice, fish, lamb, beef, pork, and green leafy vegetables.

TRACE MINERALS

Even though trace minerals are needed in our body, they are seen in trace amounts only. The researchers do not know definite functions of the trace minerals but deficiencies can definitely contribute toward health problems.

PROTEINS

Proteins, from the Greek *proteios*, meaning first, are a class of organic compounds which are present in and vital to every living cell. In the form of skin, hair, nails, cartilage, muscles, tendons and ligaments, proteins hold together, protect, and provide structure to the body of a multicelled organism. In the form of enzymes, hormones, antibodies, and globulins, they catalyze, regulate, and protect the body chemistry. In the form of hemoglobin, myoglobin and various lipoproteins, they effect the transport of oxygen and other substances within an organism.

Even though there are many amino acids, twenty-two of them are vital to carry out most of the functions listed above. Amino acids are essential for normal body function, from transmission of the genetic information to the growth and maintenance of the cells of the individual organism. Body cells are able to build their own proteins from amino acids, and carry out many essential functions by means of proteins. Proteins also serve as energy sources under certain situations.

Some of the researchers work with biochemistry and nutrition strongly believe and try to support their claims by various studies that most of the human illnesses we see are arising from nutritional deficiencies due to poor intake, poor digestion and malabsorption of proteins. Overconsumption of refined carbohydrates, saturated fats, poor intake of proteins cause to have lower immune system. Some researchers have predicted that one out of two Americans will die from the effects of cardiovascular disease (CVD). One out of four Americans will die from cancer. Immune deficiency disorders are sky-rocketting. Every second person we see suffer from either fibromyalgia or chronic fatigue syndrome or headaches. There are many studies performed on inborn errors of protein metabolism. It is the ignorance of human nutritional needs that will cause the overwhelming majority of Americans to suffer and become the victims of these afflictions. But it is sad to note that none of these researchers have any clue why so many people are suffering from this many nutritional disorders. No one thinks the reason for poor digestion, poor absorption or utilization of the nutrients are due to simple food allergies. When the allergies are removed with NAET, our patients begin to digest, absorb and assimilate nutrition from their daily diet and we see significant improvement in all of the above health disorders. After desensitization for all known allergies via NAET, people may need to supplement their foods with minimal supplements only.

It is amazing to find out how allergies can complicate our existence and take the pleasure out of living. You will be amazed to find that most headaches people suffer on a daily basis have allergies as their origins. Using the methods described in Chapter 5, you can learn to test your allergies and discover the cause of your headache now.

If you learn the testing procedures and practice at home, it won't be long before you find out that most of your health problems (including headaches) have their roots in your daily diets, clothes, other substances and products you use or come in contact with including the vitamins, other supplements, various medications and the enzymes you were using which you thought were helping you to live healthy and well.

How surprised you will be when you discover (for example) that:

Your 20-year-old migraine was due to an allergy to eggs and aggravated by eating eggs and chicken products or due to dried beans (proteins) taken to supplement your diet with enough protein?

An allergy to your soft, expensive feather pillow was causing your chronic sinusitis and early morning stuffiness and sinus headaches.

Your constant upper backache and headache at the back of the neck were due to an allergy to the pesticide that was sprayed regularly once a week in your house for years to keep the ants and roaches away.

Your daily, nagging morning headaches were due to an allergy to the smell from the coffee your husband brewed in the morning before you woke up and brought you a cup so lovingly to the bed routinely.

Your stiffneck and cluster headache were due to an allergy to the food bleach that you consumed on a daily basis via bleached white flour, white rice and white breads at most meals.

The fatigue and brain fog you experience every morning was contributed by an allergy to the diet chocolate pudding you ate at bedtime to keep your weights off and to maintain a good figure.

Your tension headaches around your menstrual cycle was due to an allergy to the tampoons and sanitary napkins you used

Your migraines around your menstrual cycle was due to an allergy to your own female hormones.

The migraine you suffered every other day was actually due to an allergy to the shellfish cocktail you sampled at least four times a week at the "happy hour" time at the hotel you worked as a waiter.

Your on-going personality disorder, behavior disorder, anger, frustration, depression, frequent headaches over the forehead and mood swings were due to an allergy to the beef jerky you snacked on frequently during the small breaks you took between your computer work.

Your unresolved bad breath, low energy and brain fog and frequent headaches that developed seven years ago after an extensive dental work were contributed by an allergy to mercury that was used in the dental filling composite put in the mouth and repeatedly came in contact with mercury by eating fish at least three times a week hoping to keep you healthy.

Your severe headaches at the back of the neck and often spread to the top of the head around your menstrual cycle was due to an allergy to the table salt you consumed at your meals to curb your salt craving around your periods.

Your chronic nagging dull headache was due to an allergy to that one glass of milk you drank every morning to maintain your bone integrity and prevent osteoporosis.

Your chronic nagging headache was due to an allergy to the detergent you used to wash your clothes.

Your eye pain and tension headaches you felt at the bilateral temples once a week were caused by an allergy to the smell of the fabric softener you used with the wash once a week to reduce the static electricity from the washed clothes.

Your child's frequent sinus headaches, sinus infections and frequent sore throat were due to an allergy to the city water he drinks in school.

Your husband's afternoon headaches were due to an allergy to the cinnamon candy bar he ate every afternoon after lunch at work.

Your watering from the eyes and headaches on the forehead and over the eyes were due to the allergy to the handsoap you used to wash your hands.

Your nausea and abdominal fullness often accompanied with migraines were due to an allergy to the baked potato you ate at lunch every day at work and the potato was bought from the nearby fast-food restaurant.

How surprised were you when your frequent migraine headaches said good-bye to you and has never returned during the past seven years soon after you were desensitized for the food additive, whiten-all (a food additive used in the restaurants on baked potatoes, salads and green salads to preserve the appearance and shelf-life).

How surprised were you when you found out the cause of your evening migraines during the summer was due to the pesticides the city sprayed on the walkways of the city park where you took a long walk every evening.

Information regarding a few important acupressure points, and NAET® energy balancing points are described in the following pages. These points and techniques, when used properly according to the accompanying instructions, might help to reduce or control your presenting acute and chronic headaches. If used properly, these points can be helpful in emergency situations with unexpected episodes of headaches.

But again I would like to make the reader aware that these are only energy balancing techniques and should not be confused with actual NAET® treatment procedures done with a trained NAET® specialist. These balancing techniques will not replace the need for a trained NAET® practitioner. These techniques alone may not be sufficient to permanently eliminate your allergies and allergy-based headaches. These procedures, when used properly as described in the following pages, will: help to improve overall health, reduce allergies and allergic reactions, help with allergy-related health problems, but will not eliminate your allergies permanently.

ABOUT NAET® TESTING

In Chapter 5, you learned to test and find your allergies using NST. You have learned to test and identify allergens in general. If you want to be healthy, you are urged to practice these testing techniques and make a habit of testing everything you suspect before exposing yourself to them. When you identify the allergens, you may be able to avoid them easily.

Most people who suffer from headaches can get their symptoms under control when they complete the NAET® basic 15-50 groups of allergens successfully. Some individuals with mild to moderate type of headache may show marked improvements after they complete just five to fifteen basic groups of allergens and begin to eat foods from those desensitized groups only. But it is to their advantage to complete the 35-50 groups of allergens before they stop the treatments. So that they would have ample of foods to eat from many food groups and life won't be so borring. If someone has severe headaches they may take more than 35 treatments. They may even needed to be desensitized for environmental agents, chemical factors, emotional imbalances, and several combinations, etc. before they can get complete freedom from their headaches.

After treating each group of allergens, after 25 hours, such item should be tested individually to be certain that the treatment has been completed. Some highly sensitive individuals may need repeated treatments on individual ingredients of the mixes (for example:egg white, egg yolk, tetracycline, feathers, etc.)

The 25 hour-food restriction should be observed on all treatments. People tend to fall out of treatments when the allergens are not avoided for 25 hours. In some cases I have observed that it is necessary to avoid the treated food allergen for 30 hours or even more. This may be due to the fact that individual has a lower level immune system, probably due to chronic illnesses.

NAET TREATMENT PLAN TO REDUCE HEADACHES

1. **NAET® desensitization treatments for all known allergens:** Check NAET allergens from the list below and have them desensitized by a well trained NAET practitioner in the given order. I cannot stress the importance of following the order of treatments, because the ingredients in the first fifteen mixtures overlap with many others below. Often desensitizing the first fifteen allergens helps clear many from the list without further treatments. So the practitioner can begin testing and treating for required combinations.

2. **Acutherapy treatments using the acutherapy points (6-2 to 6-6).** These points can be massaged once or twice a day as a routine to prevent headaches. These poitns also should be massaged at the first sign of headache, then continue every ten minutes until the headache is relieved. Drink four glasses of nonallergic water daily. Energy flows well in a well hydrated body.

3. **Self-balancing for daily foods:** After the basic fifteen, begin collecting a small portion of different foods consumed daily at each meal in a glass container and self-balance using the general balancing points given in figure 6-1. Continue self-balanc-

ing for each meal separately for a month. Then collect a small portion of each item from breakfast, lunch and dinner and whatever else you may eat during the day in a glass bottle and self-balance for this mixture at bedtime and put it away. No avoidance necessary for this food combining treatment. Start a new collection of sample on the next day and continue this procedure for a year. By doing this you will eliminate the need for NAET treatments for food combinations and adverse effects on food combining.

4. Supportive therapies and supplements: Chiropractic treatments, acupuncture, massages, hydrotherapy, laser therapy, etc. have shown good results in reducing headaches. Poor posture or poor spinal alignment can trigger neck pains, muscle spasms and headaches. Uncomfortable mattresses and pillows can result in neck pains and headaches. It is wise to get nonallergic, comfortable mattresses, bed linens and pillows to prevent headaches triggering from that source. Some people have wrong eye prescription glasses leading to eye strain and headaches. Eye glasses should be checked periodically to avoid headaches arising from wrong glasses or an allergy to glasses. Any of these supportive therapies can be used to reduce headaches while going through initial few NAET® treatments to keep the headaches under control. When most of the allergens get desensitized through NAET, other therapies can be reduced or used as needed basis.

5. Stretching of the neck muscles: This may help restricted nerve energy supply to reestablish to the brain and affected areas. Stretching at the first sign of headache is more beneficial.

Procedure: Find a comfortable chair and sit with thighs slightly apart. Bend and place your head between your thighs for five minutes. Then lift it up and hold for five minutes. Then again place between the thighs for five minutes. Repeat this cycle "five minutes between thighs, five minutes off the thighs" until you feel better.

6. Soak your feet in warm water (as hot as can be tolerated): Take a bucket and fill it half way with warm water and soak your feet in the water for an hour at a time. If the water gets cold more hot water may be added to bring up the temperature. Soaking the water in warm water will improve the energy flow in the stomach meridian and the energy will circulate freely thus helping the energy to flow from the forehead towards the feet and from there out of the meridian rendering the headache victim a great relief from headaches. Food allergy related migraines, cluster, or tension headaches can be helped this way.

6. Herbal teas to reduce headaches: Nature has invented some natural cures for devastating headaches. Most of these kitchen herbs and spices are used very effectively by many herb-lovers to find relief from headaches. A few of the commonly used herbs are given below:

Rosemary: This herb is known to be very effective for people with migraines and tension headaches since it reduces the nervous tension and eases muscular tension in tension headaches. Rosemary oil can be applied to the temples. **to make tea:** two teaspoonfull of dried leaves can be made into tea and can be taken as hot or cold tea. Should not take more than once every eight hours.

Feverfew: used very effectively by migrainers. If taken regularly, it can prevent them from happening and if they come probably with less frequency or intensity. feverfew leaf may be chewed during headaches or taken as tea. Pregnant women should not take feverfew since it is contraindicated in pregnancy.

Passionflower: This is a natural tranqueliser. it eases stress by relieving muscular and nervous tension. This is a good herb to reduce tension headaches. It can be taken as capsules, extracts, or as tea. After taking this herb, one should be carefull while driving or operating machinaries since it can cause drowsiness.

White Willow Bark: This herb is known as "herbal aspirin". It containes the active same ingredients, salicylates, as does aspirin. Aspirin is a more concentrated source of these compounds. This herb can be used as you would use aspirin, this is safer and gentle in action. **To make tea with white willow bark:** Soak one teaspoon of powdered bark in a cup of cold water for eight hours. Strain and drink as many as three cups a day. You may add honey and lemon for better taste. It is slightly bitter.

7. Maintaining adequate nutrition: The body tends to heal on its own provided it receives the right nutritional support to its vital organs. Migraine sufferers are usually deficient in certain vitamins and minerals: calcium, magnesium, vitamin B2, B6, omega-3 and omega-6 fatty acids. You should make a routine of taking adequate nonallergic multivitamin, multimineral supplements daily to maintain adequate supply of nutritients. Enegy Enfusion supplement from **www.endfatigue.com** is a good source of well researched supplement that supply adequate amount of vitamins, minerals and essential aminoacids.

We have also found supplements triggering headaches in many patients. If you take too many kinds of supplements at one time they can interact with each other producing symptoms of excess.To overcome some of these problems, we have developed a few well researched, well balanced, herbal dietary supplent to support the body function by supplying adequate essential nutrients. This formula has been found not only supplying right kind and amount of nutrients to each major meridian in the body and but have shown in reducing other health disorders related to each meridian described in Chapter four.

"ENEGY AND MORE" herbal blend is prepared from a carefully selected list of 45 adaptogenic herbs from Eastern and Western herbal pharmacy to provide all essential nutrients to each and every vital organ in the body in order to bring a harmonious balance.

Please visit the web site: www.naet.com or www.herbs2rejuve to learn more about these vital Qi balancing herbal supplements.

PREFERRED ORDER OF TREATMENTS

1. BBF (Body balance should be done before beginning NAET desensitization treatments).

2. Egg Mix (egg white, egg yolk, chicken, and tetracycline, feather.)

You may have brown or white rice, pasta without eggs, vegetables, fruits, milk products, oils, beef, pork, fish, coffee, juice, soft drinks, water, and tea.

To be checked individually: egg white, egg yolk, chicken, feather, tetracycline.

3. Calcium mix (breast milk, cow's milk, goat's milk, milk albumin, casein, coumarin, lactic acid and calcium)

You may have cooked rice, cooked fruits and vegetables (like potato, squash, green beans, yams, cauliflower, sweet potato), chicken, red meat, and drink coffee, tea without milk, and distilled or boiled, cooled water.

To be checked individually: Milk albumin, milk casein, calcium coumarin and lactic acid.

4. Vitamin C mix (fruits, vegetables, chlorophyll, bioflavonoids, vinegars, citrus, and berry. Check them individually for vitamin C supplents and all of the above ingredients in vitamin C mix.)

You may have cooked white or brown rice, pasta without sauce, boiled or poached eggs, baked or broiled chicken, fish, red meat, brown toast, deep fried food, French fries, salt, oils, coffee without milk, and water. When the vitamin C treatment is over it is advised to bring fresh green leafy vegetable and other vegetables to get checked individually and treat for them if necessary.

5. B complex (15 B-vitamins: Biotin, Choline, Inositol, PABA, Vitamin B1, Vitamin B2, Vitamin B3, Vitamin B4, Vitamin B5, Vitamin B6, Vitamin B9 (Folic acid), Vitamin B12, Vitamin B13, Vitamin B15, Vitamin B17. Check them individually.)

You may have cooked white rice, cauliflower raw or cooked, well cooked or deep fried fish, salt, white sugar, black coffee, French fries, and purified, non allergic water. Rice should be washed well before cooking. It should be cooked in lots of water and drained well to remove the fortified vitamins. After successfully completing the treatment for vitamin B-complex (should be checked for individual B vitamins, if necessarey should be treated individually), vitamin B complex should be supplemented as needed for the body or include two servings of whole grains in the daily diet.

6. **Sugar Mix** (cane sugar, corn sugar, maple sugar, grape sugar, rice sugar, brown sugar, beet sugar, fructose, molasses, honey, dextrose, glucose, and maltose.)

You may have white rice, pasta, vegetables, vegetable oils, meats, eggs, chicken, water, coffee, tea without milk. To be checked individually for all sugars.

7. **Iron Mix** (animal and vegetable sources, beef, pork, lamb, raisin, date, and broccoli.)

You may have white rice without iron fortification, sour dough bread without iron, cauliflower, white potato, chicken, light green vegetables (white cabbage, iceberg lettuce, white squash), yellow squash, distilled water and orange juice.

8. **Vitamin A** (animal and vegetable source, beta carotene, fish and shellfish.)

You may have cooked rice, pasta, potato, cauliflower, red apples, chicken, water, and coffee without milk.

To be checked individually: fish mix, shellfish mix, beta carotene.

9. **Mineral Mix** (magnesium, manganese, phosphorus, selenium, zinc, copper, cobalt, chromium, molybdenum, trace minerals)

You may use only distilled water for washing, drinking, and showering. You may eat only cooked rice, vegetables, fruits, meats, eggs, milk, coffee, and tea. No root vegetables. Check and treat magnesium alone. An allergy to magnesium can trigger headaches.

10. Water (drinking water, tap water, filtered water, city water, lake water, rain water, ocean water, and river water.)

People can react to any water. Treat them as needed and avoid the item treated. Drink boiled cooled water during 25 hours following the treatment.

11. Salt Mix (table salt, sodium and sodium chloride.)

You may use distilled water for drinking and washing, cooked rice, fresh vegetables and fruits (except celery, carrots, beets, artichokes, romaine lettuce, and watermelon) meats, chicken, and sugars.

12. Corn Mix (blue corn, yellow corn, cornstarch, cornsilk, corn syrup.)

You may eat only steamed vegetables, steamed rice, broccoli, baked chicken, and meats. You may drink water, tea and/or coffee without cream or sugar.

13. Grain Mix (wheat, gluten, gliadin, coumarin, rye, oats, millet, barley, and rice.)

You may eat vegetables, fruits, meats, milk, and drink water. Avoid all products with gluten.

To be checked for: wheat, gluten, gliadin, coumarin, corn, oats, millet, barley, rye, and rice.

14. Yeast Mix (brewer's yeast, and bakers yeast, tortula yeast, acidophilus, yogurt, and whey.)

To be individually checked: brewer's yeast, baker's yeast, whey, yogurt, and acidophilus.

You may have vegetables, egg, meat, chicken, and fish. No fruits, no sugar products. Drink distilled water.

15. Stomach acid (Hydrochloric acid.)

You may eat raw and steamed vegetables, cooked dried beans, eggs, oils, clarified butter, and milk.

16. Base (digestive juice from the intestinal tract contains various digestive enzymes: amylase, protease, lipase, maltase, peptidase, bromelain, cellulase, sucrase, papain, lactase, gluco-amylase, and alpha galactosidase.)

You may eat sugars, starches, breads, and meats.

17. Hormones (estrogen, progesterone, testosterone)

You may eat vegetables, fruits, grains, chicken, and fish.

18. Coffe, Caffiene, Chocolate (coffee, chocolate, caffeine, tannic acid, cocoa, cocoa butter, and carob, any caffienated drugs and pain relivers.)

You may consume anything that has no coffee, caffeine, chocolate and/or carob. Avoid medication with caffeine.

19. Artificial Sweeteners (Sweet and Low, Equal, Saccharine, Twin, sucralase, splenda, and Aspartame.)

You may eat anything without artificial sweeteners. Use freshly prepared items only.

At this time start collecting a small portion of different food groups from every meal and self-balance your energy for the mixture of breakfast, lunch and dinner after each meal. Please do in this fashion for a month each meal separately. Then collect breakfast, lunch and dinner (or whatever else you may eat during the day) and self-balance for this mixture at bedtime. Then next day collect the next day's meals and self-balance before going to bed. On the third day check the first day's items and if the NST is strong you may discard it. Continue to self-balance all the items from the daily meals in this fashion for a year while you continue your regular NAET with your practitioner.

21. Animal Fats (butter, lard, chicken fat, beef fat, lamb fat, and fish oil.)

You may use anything other than the above including vegetable oils.

22. Vegetable Fats and vitamin F(Oils of corn, canola, peanut, linseed, sunflower, palm, flax seed, grape seed, evening primrose, borage, wheat germ, and coconut.)

23. Spice Mix 1 (ginger, cardamom, cinnamon, cloves, nutmeg, garlic, cumin, fennel, coriander, turmeric, saffron, and mint.)

You may use all foods and products without these items.

24. Spice Mix 2 (peppers, red pepper, black pepper, green pepper, jalapeno, banana peppers, anise seed, basil, bay leaf, caraway seed, chervil, cream of tartar, dill, fenugreek, horseradish, mace, MSG, mustard, onion, oregano.)

You may eat or use all foods and food products without the above listed spices.

25. Night-shade vegetables (bell pepper, onion, eggplant, potato, okra, tomato (fruits, sauces, and drinks.)

Avoid eating these vegetables.

26. Organs mix (a particular part of the body that is involved with the disease process. For example: lung, liver, heart, spleen, large intestine, etc.)

27. Neurotransmitters: acetylcholine, nor-epinephrine, dopamine, and serotonin. Nothing to avoid.

28. Pesticides (malathion, termite control chemicals, or regular pesticides.)

Avoid meats, uncooked vegetables and fruits, grasses, trees and flowers, public areas where pesticides, ant sprays, insecticides, and other pesticides have been sprayed.

29. Alcohol (candy, ice cream, liquid medication in alcohol, and alcohol.)

Whether or not you drink alcohol, your body needs it and makes it as and when it needs it. Alcohol is made from refined starches and other forms of sugars in the body. Many people are allergic to sugar and thus alcohol.

You may eat vegetables, meats, fish, eggs, and chicken. Avoid hairspray, after shave, homeopathic remedies with alcohol.

30. Nut Mix 1 (peanuts, black walnuts, or English walnuts.)
You may eat any foods that do not contain the nuts listed above including their oils and butter.

31. Nut Mix 2 (cashew, almonds, pecan, Brazil nut, hazelnut, macadamia nut, and sunflower seeds.)

You may eat foods that do not contain the nuts listed above including their oils and butters.

32. Bacteria Mix (eat cooked foods and drink boiled cooled water)

33. Virus Mix (eat cooked foods and drink boiled cooled water)

34. Parasites (avoidance - same as bacteria mix)

You may eat anything that does not contain vegetable oils, wheat germ oil, linseed oil, sunflower oil, soybean oil, safflower oil, peanuts and peanut oil.

35. Dried Bean Mix (dried beans, vegetable proteins)

You may eat rice, pasta, vegetables, meats, eggs, and anything other than beans and bean products.

36. Amino Acids (essential amino acids: lysine, methionine, leucine, threonine, valine, tryptophane, isoleucine, and phenylalanine. Each amino acid should be checked each one and treated individually if found weak by NST)

Amino Acids (non essential amino acids: alanine, arginine, aspartic acid, carnitine citrulline, cysteine, glutamic acid, glycine, histidine, ornithine, proline, serine, taurine, and tyrosine).

You may eat cooked white rice, beef, and iceberg lettuce.

37. Food additives (sulfates, nitrates, BHT, whiten-all.)

You cannot eat hot dogs or any pre-packaged food. Eat anything made at home from scratch.

38. Food colorings (ice cream, candy, cookie, gums, drinks, spices, other foods, and/or lipsticks, and other sources.)

You may eat foods that are freshly prepared. Avoid carrots, natural spices, beets, berries, frozen green leafy vegetables like spinach.

39. Heavy metals (Lead, mercury, arsenic, antimony, zinc, cadmium, copper, siver, gold, aluminum, sulfur, vanadium and fluoride.)

Avoid tap water, green vegetables and whole grains.

40. Starch Complex (Grains, root vegetables, Carbohydrates (Avoid all type of carbohydrates).

You may have all vegetables except root vegetables, grains, yogurt, meats, chicken, and fish.

Refined starches are used as a thickening agent in sauces and drinks. Many people are allergic to starches. Refined starches should be avoided.

41. Drugs: Any drugs given in infancy, during childhood or taken by the mother during pregnancy.

Antibiotics (check Individual antibiotics), sedatives, laxatives and recreational drugs.

42. RNA, DNA, nuclear proteins and combinations.

Nothing to avoid.

43. Immunizations and Vaccinations: either you received or your parent received before you were born. Test them individually and if found treat them individually if needed.

MMR: (measles, mumps, rubella), DPT: (diphtheria, pertussis, tetanus), Polio vaccine, Small pox, Chicken pox, Influenza, hepatitis-B, hepatitis C.)

Each one of them should be checked and treated individually if tested to be an allergen. Nothing to avoid while treating for these except infected persons or recently inoculated persons if there are any near you. MMR and DPT should be treated for the individual components since allergic reactions to these vaccines are causing imbalances in the brain in many children.

44. Mercury (Avoid eating fish and all mercury products)

45. Gelatin

You may use anything that does not contain gelatin.

46. Gum Mix (Acacia, Karaya gum, Xanthine gum, black gum, sweet gum, and chewing gum).

You may eat rice, pasta, vegetables, fruits without skins, meats, eggs, and chicken; drink juice and water.

47. Baking powder/ Baking soda (in baked goods, toothpaste, and/or detergents, yogurt, cosmetics.)

Avoid any items with baking powder and baking soda. You may eat or use anything that does not contain baking powder or baking soda including fresh fruits, vegetables, fats, meat, and chicken.

48. Vitamin E, D, K

Check them individually, if needed treat them individually. You may eat fresh fish, carrots, potato, poultry, and meat.

49. Other Enzymes: Secretin, melanin, cytokinine, dopamine, histamine, endorphin, enkephalin and metabolic enzymes.

50. School work materials and **Work material** (crayons, coloring paper and books, inks, pencils, crayons, glue, play dough, other arts and craft materials, liquid paper, office work material, etc.)

Avoid using them or contacting them. Wear a pair of gloves if you have to go near them.

51. Fabrics (daily wear, sleep attire, towels, bed linens, blankets, formaldehyde, dry cleaned clothes, etc. Check individually: wool, cotton, polyester, acrylic, rayon, sofa cover, pillow cases, mattresses, crude oil, synthetic materials and products, etc.)

Treat each kind of fabric separately and avoid the particular cloth or kind of cloth for 25 hours.

52. Chemicals mix (chlorine, clorox, bleach, housecleaning products, swimming pool water, detergent, fabric softener, soap, other cleaning products, shampoos, hair products, body care products, chemicals sprays of any kind, deoderizers of any kind, lipsticks, and cosmetics you or other family members use).

Avoid the contact and smell of these chemicals for 25 hours or more as tested by your NAET practitioner. In a severely sensitive person, this treatment may need to be repeated for more than a few times to achieve complete clearance. After clearing this sample, test all other chemical items from your house or work that you are coming in contact with or you have contacted or used it in the past. Clorox is being added in various food products, herbs, spices, etc. to reduce microbial activity. This has been found one of the culprits to people who suffer from headaches as well as chemically sensitive people. Avoid everything that has clorox or bleach in them while going through the treatments. Avoid white flour, white fabrics (they all are bleached), spices and herbs prepacked by respective companies, milk, soft drinks, city water, any housecleaning products, etc.

You may eat brown rice, potato boiled with the skin (peel of the skin after boiling), cooked beef, salt, drink distilled water.

53. Plastics (toys, play or work materials, utensils, toiletries, computer key boards, plastic toys on the crib, remote control for television., alarm clock on the bedside table, and/or phone.) Avoid contact with products made from plastics during treatment. Wear a pair of cotton gloves.

54. Perfume Mix (room deodorizers, soaps, flowers, perfumes, or after-shave, etc.).

Avoid perfume and any fragrance from flowers or products containing perfume.

55. Paper Products (newspaper, newspaper ink, reading books, bills and folders, manila envelops, glues on the envelops, coloring books, books with colored illustrations).

Avoid the particular product that is treated.

56. Latex (shoe, sole of the shoe, elastic, rubber bands, and/or rubber bathtub toys.)

Avoid latex products.

57. Radiation (computer, television, microwave, X-ray, and the sun).

Avoid radiation of any kind.

58. Brain Tissue and parts of brain

Nothing to avoid.

59. Tissues and secretions (Cell filaments, Cell proteins, thyroid hormone, pituitary hormone, pineal gland, liver, urine, blood, sweat, Cerebrospinal fluid, and saliva)

Treat these items individually if needed. Avoid touching your own body. Wear a pair of gloves for 25 hours.

60. Inhalants

Environmental agents, pollens, weeds, grasses, flowers, etc.

61. Dust/ dust mites (avoid dust and dustmites. Wear a pair of glove and mask)

62. Smoking/nicotine (Avoid tobacco smoke in any form)

63. Insect Bites in infancy, childhood or in youth (bee stings, spider bites, or cockroach, etc.)

64. Allergies to people, animals and pets (children, spouse, mother, father, care takers, co-workers, cats, and dogs or other pets)

Avoid the ones you were treated for 25 hours.

65. Emotional allergies (fear, fright, frustration, anger, low self-esteem, and/or rejection, etc.)

There is nothing to avoid for emotional treatment.

66. Weather changes (wind, cold, dampness, heat, dryness, humidity). Check them individually and treat them if necessary.

Information regarding a few important acupuncture points is discussed in this chapter. They can be used to help control sensitivity reactions at any time on anyone. It is not a cure. It is going to provide temporary relief from the symptoms.

NAET® SELF-TESTING PROCEDURE

Hold, Sit and Test

This is the most simple allergy testing procedure. We teach this to our patients during patient-education class. This is very simple and our young patients love it. Children are thrilled by this procedure. They test secretly for their food, cookies, drinks, clothes, etc., before the parents get to test them with NST.

Materials Needed:

1. A sample holder (thin glass jar, test tube, or a baby food jar with a lid can serve as a sample-holder).

2. Samples of the suspected allergens.

All perishable items, liquids, foods, should be placed inside the jar, then the lid should be closed tightly so that the smell will not bother the patient. If it is a piece of fabric, toy, etc., it can be held in the hand. Severe allergens like pesticides, perfume, chemicals, other toxic products should only be self-tested by adults, never by children.

Procedure:

Place a small portion of the suspected allergen in the sample holder and hold it in your palm, touching the jar with the fingertips of the same hand for 15 to 30 minutes. If you are allergic to the item in the jar, you will begin to feel uneasy when holding the allergen, giving rise to various unpleasant allergic symptoms, or exaggerating the prior allergic symptoms. The intensity of symptoms experienced is directly related to the severity of the allergy. Since the allergen is inside the sample-holder when such uncomfortable sensations are felt, the allergen can be put away immediately and the person can wash his/her hands to remove the energy of the allergen from the fingertips. This should stop the reaction immediately. In this way, you can determine allergens and the degree of allergy easily without putting yourself in danger.

If you get frequent migraine headaches the following home procedure may help:

HOME-HELP FOR HEADACHE RELIEF

Take one to two ounces of purified water in the mouth and keep it inside the mouth and squish for five minutes then swallow the water at the end of five minutes. Repeat the procedure every ten minutes for five more times or until you find relief or until you find other help.

This procedure helps especially if any food (anything ingested) triggered the headache. When you consume allergic foods your body's defense system decides to fight the incoming allergens (the food). During the fight (allergic reaction) between your body's defense and the foods, certain toxins are produced and circulated through the body. Your saliva would also contain the same toxin. When you take a mouthfull of water (one to two ounces of water) and leave it in the mouth for five minutes, the toxin in the saliva will get diluted to the smallest concentration possible converting the water in the mouth to a very powerful homeopathic remedy towards the circulating toxin. When you drink that water it is like taking a powerful homeopathic remedy. This technique has given great relief to many migraine patients. This should arrest the headache in people if the headache is triggered from something ingested.

Some of the methods for self-balancing procedures are described in the following pages with appropriate diagrams for easy understanding. Please learn the procedure and practice to help you feel better.

GENERAL BALANCING POINTS

You may use general balancing points as shown in figure 6-1 to balance your body. These points in the order given in 6-1 can be massaged once or twice-a-day while you are going through NAET treatments with a practitioner. This will help you finish the treatments easier without having to repeat multiple times for the same allergen.

You don't have to be sick to benefit from balancing the body. You can use these balancing techniques with or without NAET® treatments. Using these points you can never overbalance the body or overtreat the meridians. One can never be too healthy.

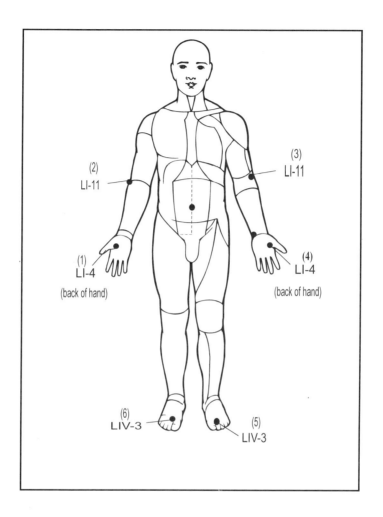

FIGURE 6-1

GENERAL BALANCING POINTS

This technique can also be used in balancing the body any time you feel out of balance. How do you know if you are out of balance? If you are a healthy person, if your energy gets slightly out of balance you may not feel sick but may not feel quite right. You may feel tired, or sleepy in the afternoon, or not having the right motivation to do your work, etc., but you cannot find a definite reason for such "out of sorts" feeling. Some minor energy disturbance in the meridians may be the cause. If you can immediately balance the body using these points, you will clear the energy blockage and feel normal in minutes.

LOCATION OF PAIN, CORRESPONDING ACUPUNCTURE MERIDIANS AND ACUPRESSURE TREATMENT POINTS

You may use these acutherapy headache reducing points as shown in figure 6-2 to 6-6 to bring relief and/or often eliminate your headaches temporarily. You should start massaging these points at the beginning of your headache for faster results. If you wait to long, you may need to massage frequently for a number repetitions before you can get relief. Select your points according to the Oriental medical category of headaches as shown below. These points can be massaged gently in the order given on the corresponding figures, one minute clockwise on each point, once every ten minutes until you feel relief.

Back of the head - Bladder meridian related headache (see figure 6-2)

Front of the head (Forehead) - Stomach meridian related (see figure 6-3)

Side(s) of the head - Gall bladder meridian related (see figure 6-4)

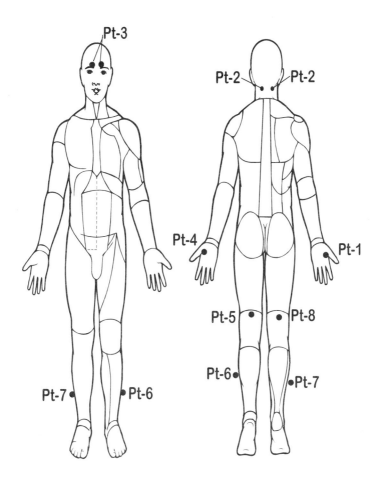

Figure 6-2

**Acutherapy points for headache
at the back of the Head**

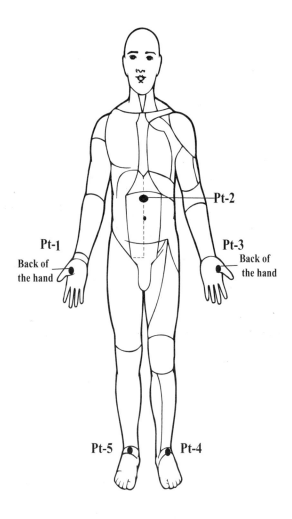

Figure 6-3

**Acutherapy points for
Frontal headache**

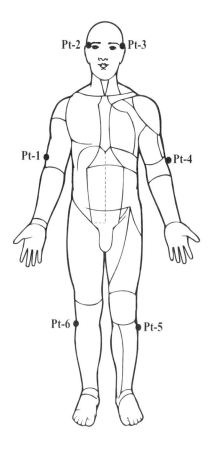

Figure 6-4

**Acutherapy points for headache
at the side(s) of the Head**

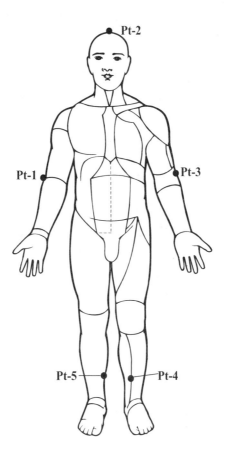

Figure 6-5

**Acutherapy points for headache
at the top of the Head**

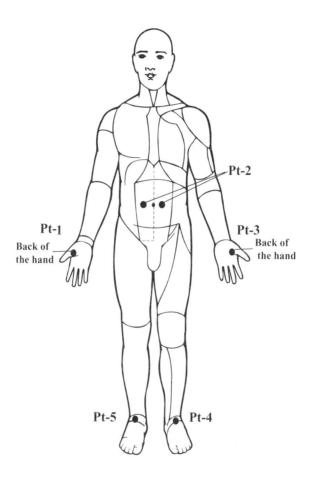

Figure 6-6

**Acutherapy points for headache
over the eyes**

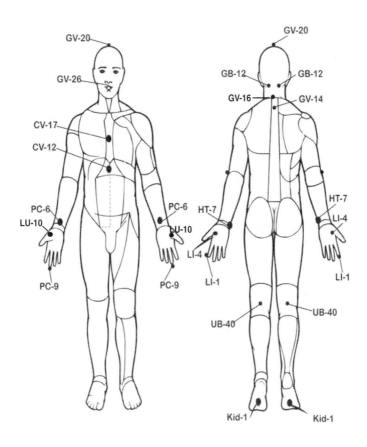

Figure 6-7

Resuscitation Points

Top of the head - Liver meridian related headache (see figure 6-5)

Eyeball(s) - Stomach and Colon meridians related headache (see figure 6-6)

Acute Care

If a person is having an acute headache, you can use general balancing points to help bring the headache under control. Using the same method described above, massage these points or emergency points often until the problem is resolved or until help arrives.

Some patients can experience physical or emotional pain or emotional release during these treatment sessions. If the patient has an emotional blockage, it needs to be isolated and treated for the best result. Some patients can get tingling pains, sharp pains, pulsation, excessive perspiration, etc. during the treatment. In such instances, please go through another cycle of treatment. Often this will correct the problem.

The Oriental Medicine CPR Point

The CPR (Cardiopulmonary rescscitation) point of Oriental Medicine is the Governing Vessel-26.

Location: Below the nose, a little above the midpoint of the philtrum.

Indication: Fainting, sudden loss of consciousness, cardiac arrhythmia, heart attack, stroke, sudden loss of energy, hypoglycemia, heatstroke, sudden pain in the lower back, general lower backache, breathing problem due to allergic reactions, mental confusion, mental irritability, anger, uncontrollable rage, exercise-induced anaphylaxis, anaphylactic reactions to allergens, and sudden breathing problem due to any cause.

Procedure: Massage or stimulate the point for 30 seconds to a minute at the beginning of the problem.

If you are treating yourself to wake up from sleeping while driving, or to recover from sudden loss of energy, etc., massage gently on this point. For example: While you are driving, if you feel sudden loss of energy or sensation of fainting, immediately massage this point. Your energy will begin to circulate faster and you will prevent a fainting episode.

For more information on revival techniques, refer to Chapter 3, pages 570 to 573, in "Acupuncture: A Comprehensive Text", by Shanghai College of Traditional Medicine, Eastland Press, 1981 or refer to "Living Pain Free with Acupressure" by the author. It is available at various bookstores and on the website (naet.com).

One or more of these emergency help points or resuscitation points can be massaged gently but firmly clockwise to help you out of emergency situations.

In Chapter four we learned about the twelve acupuncture meridians and their pathological symptoms. In Chapter 5, using "Neuromuscular Sensitivity Testing," we learned to detect the cause of energy disturbances by testing via NST. We also found that allergies may be the causative agents for most health disorders including various types of headaches. We have learned to test and find the causes of headaches in general. Practice these testing techniques and make a habit of testing for everything before exposing yourself. Make use of these self-testing and self-balancing procedures, so that you can live a normal life without headaches.

CHAPTER 7

TESTIMONIALS

NAET CHANGED THE WAY I PRACTICE MEDICINE

I'm an allopathic physician, with Residency Training in Pediatrics and extensive cross cultural and academic experience in this field for the past 14 years.

Fortunately or unfortunately, learning valuable medical experiences do not stop after formal medical training in Medical School nor Residency in any field of practice. And what I learned in these postgraduate years is that there's no single treatment modality (whether it is allopathic, chiropractic, acupuncture, psychotherapy, etc, etc…) that is going to solve one's health problem 100%. I also realized that as a regular pediatrician treating children with chronic illnesses (such as asthma, ADHD, seizure disorder, chronic otitis media/sinusitis…), I was actually not helping them to grow as healthy adults but making them chronically drug dependent adults who develops (sooner or later) new symptoms as the result of multiple pharmacotherapy, as many times physicians attempt to counteract the side effect of one drug by adding a new drug, therefore creating a vicious cycle.

I began to search new ways to treat patients and find NAET very effective because it does not only provides energetic but also material input to the treatment process using a combination of different techniques (Allopathic, Acupuncture/Acupressure, Kinesiology and Nutrition) to address an illness, each one working synergistically with each other without causing permanent side effects as pharmacotherapy often does. NAET certainly changed the way I practice Medicine today. I've been very successful using this technique in my family members and now I'm using this technique with my patients, also with positive results.

I wouldn't be so certain to tell you all this if I hadn't been a NAET patient myself. Thankfully I'm also a NAET success story after given a diagnosis of "incurable illness" not long ago. I now wake up every morning feeling thankful for having met Dr. Devi, Mala and Mohan and for having the opportunity to have learned NAET from them (I took all the Advanced Courses and worked with them at their clinic for few months in order to get a good "grasp" of MRT/NST). I can now treat myself at the convenience of my home and schedule, 4-5 times a week. I continue to improve every day.

Because of this magnificent personal experience, I decided that I wanted to develop an integrative model of care, using primarily NAET in my private practice. This is the reason I'm currently taking Medical Acupuncture Training Course at UCLA and preparing for my 4th Board Title next year. Interestingly, some physicians whom I met at UCLA come to my office to be treated with NAET for illnesses that allopathic medicine does not have much to offer other than giving diagnosis.

Medical practice evolves with time. The way we practice medicine today is not the same way it used to be practiced 50 or 100 years ago. I just hope that NAET will be a standard medical practice one day, just as acupuncture is well accepted today and taught in many reputable academic medical institutions in the United States. American medical institutions are only now learning what Chinese medical institutions knew 2000 years ago. We certainly have a lot of "catching up" to do. However, it's never too late.

As a pediatrician, UCLA trained medical acupuncturist and NAET practitioner, I plan to treat and prevent chronic illnesses and minimize side effects of pharmacotherapy so that children can achieve their full potential without the distraction of their own illnesses or the unde-sirable effects of their medications.

Respectfully,

M. Chen, MD

Diplomate of American Board of Pediatrics (1994)

Diplomate of American College of Ethical Physicians (2004)

Diplomate of American Board of Hospital Physicians (2004)

American Board of Medical Acupuncture Certification – in progress

I AM FREE OF MY INCURABLE MIGRAINES

I am a 81-year-old retired, electrical engineer. I suffered from severe migraine headaches since January 1991. I consulted various medical specialists ever since. I had many X-rays, scans, and all other possible tests to detect the cause of my headaches that came on suddenly. All the tests came negative but my headaches continued to get progressively worse. In October 2003, I was told my specialists that there is nothing much to do as treatments for my headaches except to learn to live with them. Pain pills did not give me any help even though I took them on time. I began various mild exercises including yoga, and meditation hoping to get some relief from my excrutiating headaches. I tried to eat healthy, and avoided processed foods as much as possible to avoid putting toxins into my body. I was told by some natural therapists that my body was getting toxic from living in Orange county even though I lived in Anaheim Hills that was considered a safe and healthy neighborhood. I thought I was becoming allergic to everything around me. Everything I ate, touched or breathed initiated a headache. There was nothing for me to eat or drink safely without triggering a headache. Then my wife met a lady (another customer) in a healthfood store. She told her about NAET and Dr. Devi and her wonderful permanent allergy relief treatments. She did not have Dr. Devi's phone number with her. But she remembered Dr. Devi's website: www.naet.com. We looked her up on the website. How lucky one could be! Her office was about 20 minutes from where we lived. We didn't waste anymore time. We immediately called for an appointment.When she evaluated me in her clinic, she found that my headaches were not caused by toxins from food, environmental pollution or chemical sensitivities but

Say Good-bye to Headaches

caused by certain emotional events from my past. I never believed in emotions or emotional causes triggering health problems. I thought such things only happened to weaklings. I am a German, a very brave one.

I looked at my wife who was present next to me while Dr. Devi was doing her special testing to detect the cause of my headache. She knew how I felt about emotions. She whispered into my ears, "I don't want to hear a word," she said, "You are the one suffering from headaches. Let her find out what they are from and for once don't resist her treatments. I have a strong feeling that she is going to help you, Wern"

Through her special event tracking testing procedures, Dr. Devi tracked the root cause of my headache to "fear." She further tracked the initial incident related to this particular fear to an incident that happened in 1939 at the age of "19," and related to a prison life. She also said that similar fearful incidents repeated in 1991 and 2001. I was amazed how she came up with these years and ages. She had no way of knowing what I did in 1939. When these clues were given to me I remembered what happened to me at age 19 (1939). I told her that I was a prisoner of war at 19. I was serving in German Air force. During the second world war I was taken as a POW and moved to London prison where I suffered numerous tortures and during those tortures I often thought they were going to kill me. My life hadn't started at 19 and it was going to end right there... yes, of course, that was the greatest fear I ever faced in my life. I wasn't fearful during war. But as a POW, those were the most frightening few days I spent in the prison. Even now I get nightmares when I remember those days.

Then the war stopped and I was released from the prison. I moved to America at the first chance I got and since then I lived here. I couldn't remember what happened in 1991.

Again she used her tracking procedures and helped me remember the incidents. In 1991 while I was watching the news about the air attack (Desert storm) my fear from the past (subconscious mind) took over my conscious mind for a few seconds, the terrifying past memories of the war and prison life flooded through my brain and I feared how many more innocent boys will be killed or facing my fate due to the human atrocities. Suddenly I experienced a sharp shooting pain piercing through my head which lasted for a few hours. Ever since, I continued to suffered from severe migraines (my doctors diagnosed them as migraines) almost daily without a relief. How can a common man connect an event of the past to this incurable migraine that do not respond to any medical treatment? As we always say "TIME IS THE BEST HEALER," my headaches were getting slightly better in their intensities when another similar event occured in 2001-the Iraqi-war got my subconscious mind all worked up again. My frightened subconscious mind chose to protect me with never-ending headaches so that I will not watch news about wars on television anymore.

She treated me in 2003 for the emotional fear that I experienced in 1939, then in 1991, again in 2001. My headaches diminished about 60 percent after treating for the 1939- incident. Then she made me wait for 20 minutes. When she retested my body was not ready for another NAET on the same day. My fragile mind couldn't take it anymore. So I returned to her clinic on the third day. This time Dr. Mala treated me since Dr. Devi was away. I had passed my emotional treatment for 1939. She cleared my emotional blockage of 1991. After this treatment I felt almost 90 percent relief of my headache. I was made to wait for another 20 minutes. My body did not cooperate for another treatment. So I went home and returned on the third day. I had passed the previous treatments. I was ready for more treatments. This time Dr. Devi cleared me for the fear of 2001. Complete relief of my headache was achieved when she completed the treatment for the 2001-incident. I was sent home with the instruction to avoid thinking about the past war-issues for the following 24-hours. It was hard not to think about those terrifying days. But my brilliant wife had the best suggestion: to go to Las Vegas for the weekend. We enjoyed playing slot machines. When you are at the slot machines, no past ever comes to haunt you.

I returned to the clinic after 48 hours for recheck. I had passed all the treatments. I didn't need anymore teatments. I was back to eating all my regular foods already, nothing seemed to bother me anymore. My headaches left me free and clear, once again giving me freedom to live and enjoy my life the way I wanted.

Now I am a firm believer in emotions and emotional treatments. I know now that emotions can affect anyone –stronger ones or weaklings, and they can easily make one's life not worth living anymore. I completely agree with Dr. Devi when she says that there is almost always an emotional allergy (event) in most people's health disorders. She firmly believes that if one can track that emotional event and eliminate it through NAET, most people will be living normally.

I was treated by Dr. Devi and Mala in 2003. After seven long years I still remain free of my "so called incurable migraines."   NAET IS

Say Good-bye to Headaches

AWESOME!
   Thank you Dr. Devi and Dr. Mala for helping me reclaim my life back.
   W. Dayring
   Anaheim, CA

CLUSTER HEADACHES
   I suffered from cluster headaches ever since I moved into our new house five years ago. I tried allopathic medications, Chinese herbs and homeopathic remedies without any help.
   I have had allergies all my life and have just resolved to live with them. I would break out in rashes on my face; my lips and eyes would swell and itch. The doctors would give me medications and ointments and gradually it would recede temporarily for a few minutes to a few hours. No one knew the reason. But I never had cluster headaches. I was getting treatments at one of the famous hospitals in San Diego. One day (1990) I opened the San Diego Tribune newspaper and read about Dr. Devi and NAET on the cover page. I immediately made an appointment with her. In her office she discovered, by simple muscle testing, that the built-in wood work in my house was the culprit. I was asked to bring shavings from various wood fixtures, including the kitchen cabinets, from my house. After she cleared me for the wood shavings, I did not suffer from cluster headaches anymore. For the past 17 years I have remained free of my headaches.

   Cynthia B.
   Laguna Beach, CA

BEEF & MIGRAINE
   At about 5pm today, Wednesday I started getting zig-zag lines in the side of my vision, like when I've had a migraine start to come on. This hasn't happened in years. And in the past I think it was food related. I've only had 2 or 3 full-blown migraines in my life and I've usually been able to get them to not happen completely,
   I took a Motrin 800mg and lay down for a while. The vision got better but now I have a small headache behind my eyes, and very sore in the back of my neck. What's weird is that I haven't had a headache or these symptoms for years.
   I contacted Dr. Chernoff. She evaluated me and said: Beef mix is causing the problem. Are you consuming beef daily, as in meat, fat, etc?

It's affecting your blood supply to the head and the adrenals. I was not a beef lover. I hadn't eaten beef for a long time. But I rememberd that I ate beef lately. I told her: "Monday I had steak at lunch and steak with other friends that night. And before that I cooked and ate steak twice last week."

Of course as usual, I felt great after my treatment! I woke up with no headache or neck pain. About 11 AM had a little eye headache and neck pain that lasted a short time and then nothing. And nothing since.

Paula C.
Albuquerque, New Mexico

40-YEAR-OLD MIGRAINE

I used to have severe migraines for 40 years or so. I also developed severe arthritis. I had bad psoriasis for 20 years. I also suffered from frequent bladder infections (burning urine) and interstitial cystitis for over 40 years as long as I had migraines. I suffered from mild to moderate pressure in my lower abdomen almost always. Sometimes I had intense pain in the bladder and pelvic area with urinary urgency. In such instances, I was wearing sanitary napkins to prevent getting my clothes wet.

When I went to Dr. Devi five years ago, I was in a mess. I was limping and walking with the help of a cane because my arthritis and bursitis were so bad. Dr. Devi treated me for food allergies. I was also treated for pollens, grasses and flowers. I do not have migraines anymore. My arthritis is almost 90 percent gone. Whenever I try a new food without testing, my ten percent of the arthritis returns. My psoriasis is almost gone, except for some pinpoint spots at the elbows. She found that I was very allergic to cotton and the detergent. After she cleared me for cotton and the detergent, I haven't had any bladder infection or symptoms associated with my interstitial cystitis. I have lots of energy. I walk four miles every morning. I am making up for the lost time in my youth due to pain. I don't have any pain now. I enjoy every precious day of my life now.

Maxine P.
Bellflower, CA

SINUS HEADACHES AND ALLERGIC RHINITIS

Say Good-bye to Headaches

I came to Doctor Devi a year ago with sinus headaches, shortness of breath, coughing , runny nose and wheezing. Within the first two months, my sinus headaches were reduced almost by 90 percent. The coughing and wheezing are virtually all gone. Now, we are working on eliminating allergy symptoms. I have been very pleased with her treatment and I have recommended her to many others.

Jim Ashley
Anaheim, CA

PMS and Sinus Headaches

Prior to NAET treatment, I had sinus headaches every month just before my periods that lasted four-five days after my periods started. I also suffered from frequent bouts of bronchitis and chronic low backache during those days. I also gained five to ten pounds before my periods. After treating for vitamin C mix, sugar mix, salt mix and spice mix, I do not have PMS anymore. I do not have abnormal weight gain before my periods anymore.

Colleen M.
Tustin, CA

MY SON'S MIGRAINES

My children and I started seeing Dr. Chernoff in the early part of 2000, "mainly," I told myself, "for my children's allergies." But, she has proven to be the best doctor for me also. My 15 year-old son was having chronic migraines and the medical doctors wanted to put him on increasingly stronger medication each time we went in. I didn't feel good about putting more chemicals into this boy's body, since I thought that chemicals were causing his migraines. Well, my friend had recently started seeing Dr. Chernoff and I decided to try it. She cleared his migraines, along with some allergies in just a few visits. He hasn't had a migraine . headache like that since then and he's 20 years old now.

Wanda, M.
New Mexico

258

MY HEADACHES WERE FROM MSG

I have suffered from headaches for years. Unbeknownst to me, these headaches were caused by food allergies. I used to eat Chinese food and would get sick and get a headache. After Dr. Devi treated me for MSG, I no longer suffer from any headaches when I eat Chinese food.

Linda, B.

La Mirada , CA

I AM FREE AT LAST!

If you have ever had a persistent headache or toothache, you can understand what chronic pain feels like. Chronic pain became a major part of my life a few years ago in the form of vulvodynia. This is a rare condition of the vulva that affects less than 10 percent of women and is very hard to diagnose. My pain started out as intermittent but then built up to a constant pain which rendered me unable to sit comfortably, walk, or even wear pants. It affected my ability to work and carry out a normal relationship with my boyfriend. And this also caused me to be very depressed. It took almost a year and two gynecologists to even put a name on what was causing all this pain. I had taken dozens (not an exaggeration) of prescribed of medications in order to control this pain. None of this helped. The doctor I was seeing at the time actually suggested that I have surgery to remove part of my vulva...can you imagine how painful this would be? I found this to be very insensitive advice from a man who wasn't even sure if this would put an end to this pain forever. I never considered having this surgery and I was feeling as though I was out of options. In the course of all my online research and search for others with the condition I found a reference to Dr. Marilyn Chernoff and NAET. I was willing to try anything to rid myself of this pain, so I decided to contact her. I began treatments and though it did take me a while to get to the root of my problem, I am now pain free with NO symptoms from the condition that used to render me useless. I am so happy that I found Dr. Chernoff and NAET because I am sure that without her I would still be in that pain. Dr. Chernoff has literally changed my life and I am so grateful that I can have a normal life again.

Thank you!

Jennifer S.

Say Good-bye to Headaches

Albuquerque, New Mexico

I AM FREE OF MY CHRONIC NECK PAINS

I suffered from frequent severe stiffness of the neck and upper backaches for the last 14 years. I was taking various prescriptions and over-the-counter pain pills for my neck and shoulder pain. I was told by many other doctors that it was from stress. When I was treated for spices by Dr. Devi, I was very sick during the first 18 hours after the treatment. When I woke up the next morning, I was free of my chronic neck and upper backache. It has not returned in three years.

Deborah B.
Artesia, CA

MIGRAINE AND WEATHER FORECASTING SKILL

A 60-year-old female came in with the history of migraines for over 20 years. She takes pain medication regularly whenever she got the migraines, sometimes she felt better when she took the medication, sometimes nothing helped. She suffered from headaches at least a couple of months, especially before the weather became cloudy, rainy and damp. Whenever she was down with a migraine, her family knew that they were going to have a bad weather in a few hours. I began with the basic NAET with her. When she completed her basic fifteen, she got free from her migraines. She reported lately that since she completed NAET Basics two years ago, she hasn't had a migraine. She also lost her talent in forecasting the weather.

Yumie Saito, BCSc,RN,
Shizuoka, Japan

AMAZING RECOVERY OF A STROKE PATIENT

I have had the pleasure of helping a man who had a stroke four years ago. He has also seeking care from a D.O. Neurologist (who also does NAET), Johns-Hobkins, a Naturopath, a homeopathist and a PT. The D.O. is in Tacoma, Washington and the lead on this case. When the patient initially entered my office his face was plastic like. He showed no emotion. He could not speak in sentences. He had heavy braces on his left leg. He left arm was also severely damaged by the stroke.

We cleared the basics. He had a difficult time clearing copper. When Johns-Hobkins changed his copper supplement his blood pressure went up. After treating for the new copper supplement his blood pressure returned to normal. We use normal NAET protocol on him.. The patient is an attorney. He has recovered enough that the Oregon Bar is allowing him to do some pro bono work for the aged. He now has expression in his face and voice. He has also exhibited emotions. His wife attributes much of the his successes to date to his NAET treatments.

Anthony DeSiena, D.C.
Portland, Oregon

CHRONIC SINUSITIS & HEADACHES

After the (caesarean) birth of my second child, I constantly "did not feel well". I was diagnosed as having developed allergies to dust and mold. My problem was not only severe sinus headaches, but severe post nasal drip that when started was a "faucet" that could not be turned off. After being on several prescription antihistamines and nose sprays for a couple of years, nothing seemed to work. My allergist started me on allergy shots to build up my immunity. I pursued these shots for 8 years along with the antihistamines and nose sprays. Still my symptoms seemed to get more severe. For two weeks in the spring and then again in the fall, my post nasal drip was so relentless that I would end up with an upper respiratory infection and laryngitis. Not only would I have to go on antibiotics to clear up the infection, but I would have to get a steroid shot to calm down the inflammation.

I tried acupuncture and a variety of homeopathic remedies on the subject of allergies. My allergies weren't "seasonal" as it seemed for most allergy sufferers. I had more bad days than good year round. My allergist suggested I see an Ear, Nose and Throat specialist. He put me on nasal steroid shots. This helped a bit, but still twice a year I had my "episodes" that ended with the same results. I continued these shots for 4 years, constantly reading anything I could find related to allergies.

There was an article in a magazine on people with "environmental allergies". They were affected by changes in seasons, temperature, climates, humidity, barometric pressure, etc. No wonder it seemed to me like I was allergic to everything, I was! I live in NJ where 30° temperature changes in 24 hours are not uncommon. I could not wait to discuss this with my Dr. He was fully aware of this condition and advised me to move to the Southwest desert where the climate is stable year round!

After 23 years of various specialists, not only was I the one to figure out what my problem was, but was told there was no treatment that would alleviate my symptoms, outside of moving. I could not believe it but resigned myself to living with it.

My husband and I heard about NAET briefly on the news. It seemed so "hoaky" but he encouraged me to give it a try. It did not take me long to have a major breakthrough. I started in the spring. My third visit I was well into one of my "episodes" and had been sick for days. I was treated for calcium and on my ride home, I thought I could feel my post nasal drip stopping! I thought for sure it was my imagination. My husband assured me it was. By the next morning, it HAD stopped and I was feeling like I had been on antibiotics for 3 days! After Mira treated the basics, it amazed me that I could be treated for hot, cold, humidity, temperature change, etc. We then did most of the pollens, but had to stop until the next frost.

I have since gone through one fall and spring season without an "episode". I occasionally have minor symptoms but far and few apart. They are ALL good days now. I will resume treatments in the fall. I am eternally grateful to both Dr.Devi and my wonderful practitioner Mira Champaniera.

S. Miller, New Jersey
NAET Sp: Mira Champaniera

FORMALDEHYDE SENSITIVITY
A 70-year old female came in with severe migraine since two days. She tried to get medical help with her medical doctor. for the last two days. Not only she got any relief from the medication she took, she couldn't sleep for the last 48 hours or so either. In my office I used the NAET Acute care protocol to detect the cause of her headache and found out it was from some chemical she inhaled from her surroundings constatly. Then she told me that she was remodelling the house and there was paint and formaldhyde smell everywhere. It was the formaldehyde. I treated for formaldhyde energy first, then treated for the smell of formaldehyde. In less than 30 minutes she got complete relief from her migraines. I saw her again after a week. She did not have anymore headaches.

Yoshitastu Takamori, LAc, LMT
Osaka, Japan

NAET GOT RID OF MY HEADACHES

Having a severe headache is like walking a thin line between life and death. You know you're alive, you're breathing and able to communicate with others, but you're secretly wishing it could all be over, even if it results in your death. The pain is so extreme, you don't know what to do. The drugs don't help, and nothing can calm you. I remember I used to stand over the bathroom sink, expecting my nose to detach from my face because the pressure was so strong. It would blur my vision and dull my hearing and immediately, my body would go into evacuation mode. I would get tremors, diarrhea, and nausea. The doctors gave me everything from Ativan to Codeine to Valium. Nothing worked. For 2 months I took 800 mg of Motrin every 3 and 1/2 hours, and finally I felt some relief. My weight had gone from 127 pounds to 95 pounds in under two months. I was almost invisible.

When you're sick and no one can tell you what the cause or the solution is, you become increasingly hopeless. When you're ill for a long period of time, your being becomes a gas tank filled with hope. When you have countless rough days and nights, your "hope tank" becomes less full, eventually falling on empty. You don't want to continue, and you beg God to just put you out of your misery, because you're sure you can't take even one more day.

When the headaches finally stopped, it was like I was given a new lease on life. I was thankful for everything, even for the other symptoms that remained, because the other symptoms caused a different kind of pain, and I was getting a break. Your "hope tank" starts to feel full again, and you revert back to your old self, fighting to get better. Just having one good day, among many bad ones, is enough to pump more hope into your life, restoring the human spirit and its love for life. Having one bad day, pulls you back down into a pit of hopelessness, sure that you will die from whatever it is that is causing all the misery, sure that no one knows why you're sick or how to make you whole again.

Leslie B.
NAET Sp: Chernoff, ND, Ph.D.
Albuquerque, NM

Say Good-bye to Headaches

IT WAS THE BAMBOO SHOOTS

A 50-year-old female came in around 7:00 pm with the complaints of a severe headache since this morning, started after breakfast. She tried to go to work but due to the severity of the headache she couldn't go too far. So she stopped at her family physician. He gave her an injection. In the past she had received relief from injections, but today she didn't get any relief. So by 12 noon she went another doctor. He also gave her some medicine without any relief. Finally by 7:00 pm when her husband came home from work, he brought her to my office.

She looked very sick and lethargic. She said in spite of taking all the medication, her headache is getting worse by the minute. She couldn't even move her head due to extreme pain.

I couldn't perform any physical exam on her because any little movement gave her shooting pains in her head. So I used a surrogate to test her NST. With my QRT, I found out that she ate some food last night for supper and then again she ate it this morning that caused her this headache. She said she prepared bamboo shoots last night and she ate it last night and this morning. She also said since it was the season for bamboo shoots, she bought a large bunch and made lots of different dishes with it even though she ate only one kind last night and this morning. Rest of the dishes she saved them in the freezer for future use. I had no sample of bamboo shoot available in my office, so I asked her husband to get it. He returned with bamboo shoots in a few minutes. I had to desensitize her with NAET for bamboo shoots every ten minutes for three times consecutively. After the third treatment, she suddenly got up from the treatment table and said, "Oh, My God! My headache is gone!" By 8:30 pm, she left my office with a big smile on her face.

Yumie Saito, BCSc., RN
Shizuoka, Japan

IRON PILL AND CERVICALGIA

A 30-year-old female came in for chiropractic adjustment almost daily for the several days (5 days to be exact) for her neck and upper backache (Cervicalgia) and facial pain on her left side. Soon after the adjustments, she felt better and went home, only to return next day again with stiff neck, upper back and headache. On her fourth visit, I was puzzled about her repeated nerve impinchment. I tested her using QRT and found out that she was allergic to iron and she was taking it in a prescription form to help with her anemia. I treated her for her prescription iron pill and she did not get anymore neckpains and headaches when she took those pills again.

Yoshihito Tatebe, LMT
Yokohama, Japan

AFLATOXIN INDUCED HEADACHE

A 30-year-old male suffered from frequent daily cluster headaches for the past three months. He tried various treatments both from allopathic and holistic methods during the past three months without any relief. Finally suggested by one of his co-workers from his company, he came to see me. He was fairly healthy up until three months ago when he began his unique daily occurrances of headaches. I tested using NAET-QRT method and detected that his headaches were from something he ate on a regular basis for the past three months. Upon questioning he said he had bought a large container of peanuts three months ago since he found them on sale and he was eating a handfull of them everyday. It was the peanuts, especially the aflatoxins produced by the peanut mold. The peanut was already old when he bought them on a discounted price and probably the mold began releasing toxins into the nuts. I treated him for aflatoxin and he got freed of his headaches in the next few hours.

Hiroshi Masuda, DC, DACNB
Shizuoka, Japan

END OF MY EXPLOSIVE HEADACHES

Thank you! Dr. Marilyn for coming to my rescue when I needed your help most. On two occasions I have had an explosive headache and fatigue. You detected the problem and treated the pain. I would not have believed it if I didn't experience it myself?

Say Good-bye to Headaches

On December 30, 2001, I suffered an incredible explosive headache. It was so bad that I asked my husband to take me to the emergency room. I thought my head would literally explode! You treated the pain for a strep and viral infection. The next day I felt great! Unbelievable!

On January 12, 2002, I had a shooting right side headache. My right eye felt like someone was piercing it! I was tired and dizzy. I had picked up two viruses at the school where I taught Special Education. Thirty minutes after the treatment, my husband came in and asked how I was doing? I said that my headache went away. I rested that afternoon and evening. The whole treatment took about 24 hours. The next day I was back to myself again – no headache, dizziness or fatigue –the viruses were gone? Amazing? I have never experienced anything like this before. Each time you treat me, I seem to get better and better overall health in addition to ridding the virus or infection!!!

I use to have to see a chiropractor at least once a week to straighten my back and neck. Since working with Dr. Marilyn I do not have to visit one anymore.

Louise Swartswalter
Albuquerque, NM
NAET Sp: Marilyn Chernoff, ND., Ph.D.

ALLERGY TO THE NEW BATCH OF TABLE SALT

A 65-year-old woman also came in with severe right sided migraine. She was allergic to the new batch of salt she bought a couple of days ago. Soon after she was treated for the new salt, her migraine said good-bye to her within the next ten minutes.

Yumie Saito, BCSc., RN
Shizuoka, Japan

Glossary

Abdominal Migraine - A type of migraine that mainly occurs in childhood, characterized by abdominal pain, nausea, vomiting, and sometimes diarrhea, but with little or no headache. Later in life, children with abdominal migraine may develop more typical migraine attacks.

Abortive Medication - Medication taken to "abort" or stop a headache after it already begins.

Acetaldehyde: An aldehyde found in cigarette smoke, vehicle exhaust, and smog. It is a metabolic product of Candida albicans and is synthesized from alcohol in the liver.

Acetaminophen - An aspirin substitute. Like aspirin, acetaminophen works as a pain killer and fever reducer, but it does not have anti-inflammatory properties and does not produce the side effects associated with aspirin, such as stomach irritation.

Acetylcholine: A neurotransmitter manufactured in the brain, used for memory and control of sensory input and muscular output signals.

ACHE - American Council for Headache Education, an organization affiliated with AHS, and made up of both headache patients and professionals who treat headache. The purpose of the organization is to educate patients and the public about headache, and to advocate up-to-date treatment for headache sufferers.

Acid: Any compound capable of releasing a hydrogen ion; it will have a pH of less than 7.

Acupressure - Derived from traditional Chinese medicine, this is a form of treatment for pain that involves pressure on particular points in the body know as "acupressure points".

Acupuncture - Derived from traditional Chinese medicine, this is a form of treatment for pain that involves insertion of fine needles into particular points in the body known as "acupuncture points".

Say Good-bye to Headaches

Acute: Extremely sharp or severe, as in pain, but can also refer to an illness or reaction that is sudden and intense.

Adaptation: Ability of an organism to integrate new elements into its environment.

Addiction: A dependent state characterized by cravings for a particular substance if that substance is withdrawn.

Additive: A substance added in small amounts to foods to alter the food in some way.

Adrenaline: Trademark for preparations of epinephrine, which is a hormone secreted by the adrenal gland. It is used sublingually and by injection to stop allergic reactions.

AHS - American Headache Society, a professional organization of physicians, dentists, physician's assistants, nurses, and other health professionals and scientists interested in the study of headache and its' treatment.

Aldehyde: A class of organic compounds obtained by oxidation of alcohol. Formaldehyde and acetaldehyde are members of this class of compounds.

Alkaline: Basic, or any substance that accepts a hydrogen ion; its pH will be greater than 7.

Allergenic: Causing or producing an allergic reaction.

Allergen: Any organic or inorganic substance from one's surroundings or from within the body itself that causes an allergic response in an individual is called an allergen. An allergen can cause an IgE antibody mediated or non-IgE mediated response. Some of the commonly known allergens are: pollens, molds, animal dander, food and drinks, chemicals of different kind like the ones found in food, water, inside and outside air, fabrics, cleaning agents, environmental materials, detergent, cosmetics, perfumes, etc., body secretions, bacteria, virus, synthetic materials, fumes of any sort, including pesticide fumes, fumes from cooking, etc., and smog. Emotional unpleasant thoughts like anger, frustration, etc. can also become allergens and cause allergic reactions in people.

Glossary

Allergic reaction: Adverse, varied symptoms, unique to each person, resulting from the body's response to exposure to allergens.

Allergy: Attacks by the immune system on harmless or even useful things entering the body. Abnormal responses to substances that are usually well tolerated by most people.

Amino acid: An organic acid that contains an amino (ammonia-like NH3) chemical group; the building blocks that make up all proteins.

Amitriptlyine - An anti-depressant medication useful in treating migraine and tension type headaches.

Analgesic - Medication for the relief of pain. An analgesic works to increase the patient's pain threshold, thereby decreasing the sensation of pain. Analgesics range from aspirin and acetaminophen to narcotics.

Anaphylactic shock: Also known as anaphylaxis. Usually happens suddenly when exposed to a highly allergic item. But sometimes, it can also happen as a cumulative reaction. (first two doses of penicillin may not trigger a severe reaction, but the third or fourth could produce an anaphylaxis in some people). An anaphylaxis (this life threatening allergic reaction) is characterized by: an immediate allergic reaction that can cause difficulty in breathing, light headedness, fainting, sensation of chills, internal cold, severe heart palpitation or irregular heart beats, pallor, eyes rolling, poor mental clarity, tremors, internal shaking, extreme fear, angio neurotic edema, throat swelling, drop in blood pressure, nausea, vomiting, diarrhea, swelling anywhere in the body, redness and hives, fever, delirium, unresponsiveness, or sometimes even death.

Aneurysm - A congenital weak point in the wall of an artery that may bulge outwards, and may occasionally rupture and bleed, causing what is called a "subarachnoid hemorrhage", which produces a severe headache and stiff neck and sometimes can be fatal.

Antibody: A protein molecule produced in the body by lymphocytes in response to a perceived harmful foreign or abnormal substance as a defense mechanism to protect the body.

Say Good-bye to Headaches

Antigen: Any substance recognized by the immune system that causes the body to produce antibodies; also refers to a concentrated solution of an allergen.

Antihistamine: A chemical that blocks the reaction of histamine that is released by the mast cells and basophils during an allergic reaction. Any substance that slows oxidation, prevents damage from free radicals and results in oxygen sparing.

Anti-inflammatory - A class of drugs that reduces inflammation in the body, and that are often used to treat arthritis. These drugs can also be useful in reducing the inflammation associated with certain types of headaches, but may cause gastrointestinal upset.

Anticonvulsant - A class of drugs used to treat convulsive seizures, or epilepsy. Some of these medications, such as Valproic Acid or Depakote, are also used in prevention of headache, even when headaches are not associated with seizures.

Antidepressant - A class of drugs used primarily to treat depression. Some of these drugs have also been found to be useful in the prevention of headache, even when headaches are not associated with depression.

Antiemetics - A class of drugs used to treat nausea and/or vomiting.

Aspartame - Artificial sweetener known to act as a migraine trigger in some vulnerable people.

Assimilate: To incorporate into a system of the body; to transform nutrients into living tissue.

Autoimmune: A condition resulting when the body makes antibodies against its own tissues or fluid. The immune system attacks the body it inhabits, which causes damage or alteration of cell function.

Aura - The warning symptoms, usually visual, that may sometimes occur shortly before a migraine headache begins. The word "aura" comes from the Greek word for wind, and just as a strong wind may precede a storm, an aura may precede the storm of migraine. Auras may occur without head pain.

Barbiturate - A class of drugs that causes sedation and relaxation. Barbiturates may be found in combination abortive medications used to treat the symptoms of headache. If used too frequently (more than a couple of days per week), they may be habit-forming.

Basilar Migraine - A type of migraine that mainly affects children and adolescents. Associated with the headache are a number of symptoms related to the part of the brain supplied by the basilar artery. These include vertigo (spinning sensations), loss of balance, and sometimes, loss of consciousness as well as prominent nausea and vomiting.

Benzodiazepines - A category of potentially addictive tranquilizers that may increase depression at the same time that they reduce anxiety.

Beta Blockers - A class of drugs used to treat heart disease and high blood pressure. These drugs lower blood pressure and slow the heart rate. They were discovered accidentally to also be useful for preventing migraine headaches.

Biofeedback - A form of treatment for headache that uses electronic feedback of hand temperature and/or muscle tension to rapidly teach patients how to deeply relax. Acquiring and regularly practicing these skills has been shown to often reduce the frequency and severity of both migraine and tension-type headaches.

Binder: A substance added to tablets to help hold them together.

Blood brain barrier: A cellular barrier that prevents certain chemicals from passing from the blood to the brain.

Buffer: A substance that minimizes changes in pH (Acidity or alkalinity).

Caffeine - A stimulating drug found in coffee, tea, and cola beverages. After a headache begins, caffeine may be helpful in aborting headaches, so it is widely used in combination drugs prescribed for relief of headache. Paradoxically, using caffeine to excess or too rapid withdrawal from caffeine, may cause headaches in some individuals.

Caffeine Withdrawal Headache - A headache caused by dilation of the blood vessels once the constrictive effects of caffeine are no longer present.

Calcium Channel Blocker - A type of medication that may prevent migraine headaches by acting on the blood vessels, the brain, or both.

Say Good-bye to Headaches

Candida albicans: A genus of yeast like fungi normally found in the body. It can multiply and cause infections, allergic reactions or toxicity.

Candidiasis: An overgrowth of Candida organisms, which are part of the normal flora of the mouth, skin, intestines and vagina.

Carbohydrate, complex: A large molecule consisting of simple sugars linked together, found in whole grains, vegetables, and fruits. This metabolizes more slowly into glucose than refined carbohydrate.

Carbohydrate, refined: A molecule of sugar that metabolizes quickly to glucose. Refined white sugar, white rice, white flour are some of the examples.

Catalyst: A chemical that speeds up a chemical reaction without being consumed or permanently affected in the process.

CAT Scan - "Computerized Axial Tomographic" scan, a type of X-ray scan utilized for diagnostic purposes which can be useful in identifying causes of headache that may masquerade as migraine.

Cerebral allergy: Mental dysfunction caused by sensitivity to foods, chemicals, environmental substances, or other substances like work materials etc.

Chiropractic - A philosophic system of mechanical therapeutics that associates many diseases on poor alignment of the vertebrae. Chiropractors treat disease with manipulation of the vertebrae in order to relieve pressure on the nerves, "so that nerve force may flow freely from the brain to the rest of the body".

Chlorpromazine - A powerful major tranquilizer that relieves the pain and nausea of migraine.

Chronic Headache - Headache that occurs frequently over a period of time, generally at least every other day or 15 days per month for a period of at least six months.

Chronic: Of long duration.

Chronic fatigue syndrome: A syndrome of multiple symptoms most commonly associated with fatigue and reduced energy or no energy.

Classic Migraine - An older term for what is now called "migraine with aura" (see definition of aura above).

Cluster Headache - A particular type of headache that mainly affects men by a 6 to 1 ratio. It is characterized by intense but brief (30 minutes to 2 hours) pain in and around one eye occurring daily or several times per day in "clusters" that typically last for a couple of months. The patient then may go for many months with no headaches at all. Along with the headache, there are usually other phenomena such as tearing and redness of the affected eye, or stuffy nose.

Cognitive Behavioral Therapy - An approach to psychotherapy that helps patients take control of their illness, and their lives, through insight, self knowledge and planning.

Common Migraine - An older term for what is now called "migraine without aura" (see definition of aura above).

Chronic Paroxysmal Hemicrania - (CPH) A very rare headache syndrome which can resemble cluster headache as it presents itself as multiple, short, severe headaches that occurs on a daily basis. They can also be associated with tearing, nasal stuffiness, etc. CPH differs from cluster headache in that the patients are almost always female, the headache attacks are shorter (1-2 minutes) and much more frequent with attacks occurring on average of 14 times per day. This condition responds almost 100% of the time to treatment with Indomethacin.

Cumulative reaction: A type of reaction caused by an accumulation of allergens in the body.

Cytokine Immune system's second line of defense. Examples of cytokines are interleukin 2 and gamma interferon.

Daily Headache - Headache that occurs either daily or almost daily, at least 20 days per month.

Depression - Not just temporary or situational sadness, but a persistent and pervasive feeling of sadness or hopelessness that is often associated with weight loss (or gain), sleep disturbances, constipation, disturbances of sexual function, and feelings of guilt or self-blame.

Desensitization: The process of building up body tolerance to allergens by the use of extracts of the allergenic substance.

Detoxification: A variety of methods used to reduce toxic materials accu-mulated in body tissues.

Dexamethasone - A steroid drug used to treat inflammation.

Say Good-bye to Headaches

DHE - Abbreviation for Dihydroergotamine, a drug used, usually by injection or nasal spray, to treat migraine, rebound and cluster headaches.

Diagnosis - The process of taking a history and performing an examination in order to decide what is causing a particular symptom, such as headache, so that a correct treatment can be chosen.

D.O. - Abbreviation for a doctor of osteopathy, a degree indicating medical training approximately the same as that for a doctor of medicine or M.D. Practitioners of osteopathy or osteopaths, use the diagnostic and therapeutic measures of ordinary medicine in addition to having training in manipulative measures.

Dopamine - One of several chemicals called "neurotransmitters" that transmit or send messages from one nerve cell to another in the nervous system.

Digestive tract: Includes the salivary glands, mouth, esophagus, stomach, small intestine, portions of the liver, pancreas, and large intestine.

Disorder: A disturbance of regular or normal functions.

Dust: Dust particles from various sources irritate sensitive individual causing different respiratory problems like asthma, bronchitis, hayfever like symptoms, sinusitis, and cough.

Dust mites: Microscopic insects that live in dusty areas, pillows, blankets, bedding, carpets, upholstered furniture, drapes, corners of the houses where people neglect to clean regularly.

Dysrhythmia - A disturbance in the normal pattern of brain waves as recorded in encephalography (EEG). Dysrhythmias of different kinds may show up during migraine, sleep, overexcitement, etc.

Eczema: An inflammatory process of the skin resulting from skin allergies causing dry, itchy, crusty, scaly, weepy, blisters or eruptions on the skin. skin rash frequently caused by allergy.

Edema: Excess fluid accumulation in tissue spaces. It could be localized or generalized.

EEG - Electroencephalography is a test used to detect and record the electrical activity generated by the brain.

Electromagnetic: Refers to emissions and interactions of both electric and magnetic components. Magnetism arising from electric charge in motion. This has a definite amount of energy.

Elimination diet: A diet in which common allergenic foods and those suspected of causing allergic symptoms have been temporarily eliminated.

Endocrine: refers to ductless glands that manufacture and secrete hormones into the blood stream or extracellular fluids.

Endocrine system: Thyroid, parathyroid, pituitary, hypothalamus, adrenal glands, pineal gland, gonads, the intestinal tract, kidneys, liver, and placenta.

Endogenous: Originating from or due to internal causes.

Environment: A total of circumstances and/or surroundings in which an organism exists. May be a combination of internal or external influences that can affect an individual.

Environmental illness: A complex set of symptoms caused by adverse reactions of the body to external and internal environments.

EMG - Electromyography is a test used to discover diseases of the muscles, spinal cord, and peripheral nerves.

Endorphins - Hormone-like substances produced in the brain that have analgesic properties.

Episodic - Describing occurrences that come and go, with or without a regular pattern.

Ergotamine - A drug originally derived from the ergot fungus that constricts blood vessels and has been used since the 1920's to treat migraine headaches.

Exercise - Many headache specialists believe that regular physical exercise can reduce the frequency and severity of headaches, although, not many research studies have been done to prove or disprove this widespread belief. If true, exercise may help by reducing stress.

Feverfew - An herb (plant of the chrysanthemum family) used for the prevention of migraine headaches. It is more widely used in England than in this country. Potency varies from one preparation to another since this herb is not regulated by the Federal Food and Drug Administration. There are anecdotal reports in the medical literature that it is helpful, but no carefully controlled scientific studies.

"Fight" or "flight": The activation of the sympathetic branch of the autonomic nervous system, preparing the body to meet a threat or challenge.

Food addiction: A person becomes dependent on a particular allergenic food and must keep eating it regularly in order to prevent withdrawal symptoms.

Food grouping: A grouping of foods according to their botanical or biological characteristics.

Glaucoma - An eye disease that can eventually cause blindness. Glaucoma is sometimes the cause of headache pain.

Hangover Headache - A headache linked to the consumption of alcohol, which dilates and irritates the brain's blood vessels.

Head Trauma - Injury to the head, which may in some cases lead to what are called "post-traumatic headaches".

Headache - Generally refers to a persistent or lasting pain in the head region, as contrasted with a "head pain", such as trigeminal neuralgia, which is quite brief.

Histamine: A body substance released by mast cells and basophils during allergic reactions, which precipitates allergic symptoms.

Holistic: Refers to the idea that health and wellness depend on a balance between the physical (structural) aspects, physiological (chemical, nutritional, functional) aspects, emotional and spiritual aspects of a person.

Homeopathic: Refers to giving minute amounts of remedies that in massive doses would produce effects similar to the condition being treated.

Homeopathy - The practice of the use of active ingredients in minute dosages along with naturally occurring substances in order to provide a healthier balance of internal chemistry. These minute dosages would be viewed in traditional medicine as ineffective.

Hormone Replacement Therapy - The therapeutic use of synthetic hormones, usually estrogen and progesterone after menopause or following a hysterectomy.

Hormones - Powerful substances secreted by the endocrine glands in the body that are carried through the blood stream to have effects on other parts of the body distant from where they are produced.

Hydrocephalus - An uncharacteristic swelling in the amount of cerebrospinal fluid within the skull, causing dangerous expansion of the cerebral ventricles.

Hypertension Headache - A headache that strikes people who have very high blood pressure. Its "hatband" type pain can be most severe in the morning.

Hypnosis - A sleep-like state usually induced by another person in which the subject retains awareness of the presence of the hypnotist and where the subject is susceptible to heightened suggestibility. After training by a hypnotist, some migraine patients can be taught to hypnotize themselves in order to reduce stress and related symptoms.

Hypothyroidism: A condition resulting from under-function of the thyroid gland.

IgA: Immunoglobulin A, an antibody found in secretions associated with mucous membranes.

IgD: Immunoglobulin D, an antibody found on the surface of B-cells.

IgE: Immunoglobulin E, an antibody responsible for immediate hypersensitivity and skin reactions.

IgG: Immunoglobulin G, also known as gammaglobulin, the major antibody in the blood that protects against bacteria and viruses.

IgM: Immunoglobulin M, the first antibody to appear during an immune response.

Immune system: The body's defense system, composed of specialized cells, organs, and body fluids. It has the ability to locate, neutralize, metabolize and eliminate unwanted or foreign substances.

Immunocompromised: A person whose immune system has been damaged or stressed and is not functioning properly.

Say Good-bye to Headaches

Immunity: Inherited, acquired, or induced state of being, able to resist a particular antigen by producing antibodies to counteract it. A unique mechanism of the organism to protect and maintain its body against adversity by its surroundings.

Inflammation: The reaction of tissues to injury from trauma, infection, or irritating substances. Affected tissue can be hot, reddened, swollen, and tender.

Idiopathic - Occurring spontaneously, not traceable to a direct cause.

Indomethacin - A nonsteroidal anti-inflammatory medication which can be effective for the relief of migraine and other types of headaches.

Imitrex - Brand name for Sumatriptan, a fairly new migraine abortive medication available as a self-administered injection or as a tablet.

Inhalant: Any airborne substance small enough to be inhaled into the lungs; eg., pollen, dust, mold, animal danders, perfume, smoke, and smell from chemical compounds.

Intolerance: Inability of an organism to utilize a substance.

International Headache Society - An international professional organization of physicians and other health professionals and scientists interested in the study of headache and its' treatment. In 1988, the International Headache Society, or IHS, developed definitions of the different types of headaches that are widely accepted by physicians and others who treat headache world-wide.

Intractable Migraine - A migraine headache that "just won't stop". By definition, any migraine that persists longer than 72 hours is referred to as "status migrainosus". Migraines may often become transformed into a chronic daily headache by too frequent use of either painkillers or ergots.

Kinesiology: Science of movement of the muscles.

Latent: Concealed or inactive.

Leukocytes: White blood cells.

Letdown Migraine - Migraine may often occur after times of stress, as after a big exam, or on weekends after a hectic week at work. These are referred to as "letdown" attacks.

Light Sensitivity - People with migraine may become very sensitive to light, a condition known as "photophobia", or literally "fear of light". A similar sensitivity to sound may also occur, and is known as "phonophobia".

Lipids: Fats and oils that are insoluble in water. Oils are liquids in room temperature and fats are solid.

Lymph: A clear, watery, alkaline body fluid found in the lymph vessels and tissue spaces. Contains mostly white blood cells.

Lymphocyte: A type of white blood cell, usually classified as T-or B-cells.

Macrophage: A white blood cell that kills and ingests microorganisms and other body cells.

Masking: Suppression of symptoms due to frequent exposure to a substance to which a person is sensitive.

Mast cells: Large cells containing histamine, found in mucous membranes and skin cells. The histamine in these cells are released during certain allergic reactions.

Mediated: Serving as the vehicle to bring about a phenomenon, eg., an IgE-mediated reaction is one in which IgE changes cause the symptoms and the reaction to proceed.

Membrane: A thin sheet or layer of pliable tissue that lines a cavity, connects two structures, selective barrier.

Metabolism: Complex chemical and electrical processes in living cells by which energy is produced and life is maintained. New material is assimilated for growth, repair, and replacement of tissues. Waste products are excreted.

Migraine: A condition marked by recurrent severe headaches often on one side of the head, often accompanied by nausea, vomiting, and light aura. These headaches are frequently attributed to food allergy.

Magnesium - An element found in trace amounts in the body, in certain foods, and believed to possibly play a role in the cause of migraine headaches, according to some recent research.

MAO Inhibitors - Monoamine Oxidase Inhibitors are a class of drugs used for treating depression and also have been found useful in treatment of migraine. Persons taking MAO inhibitors may not eat certain foods containing tyramine because of the danger of increase in blood pressure and, therefore, must be closely monitored during treatment.

Massage - A method of manipulation of the body by rubbing, pinching, kneading, tapping, etc., that can be helpful in producing relaxation.

M.D. - Abbreviation for "medical doctor".

Menstrual Migraine - The terms "pure menstrual migraine" or "true menstrual migraine" refers to migraine attacks that occur only with menses. If attacks occur mainly but not exclusively with menses, this may be referred to as "mainly menstrual migraine".

Migraine - A particular form of recurrent headache that often runs in families. According to the International Headache Society, migraine headache pain must have four of the following characteristics: one-sided, pulsating or throbbing, at least moderate if not severe, and worsened by ordinary daily activities such as climbing stairs or housework. In addition, the pain must be accompanied by either nausea or else sensitivity to light and noise. There must be no evidence of other disease and at least 4-5 attacks before a physician can be confident of the diagnosis.

Migraine Equivalents - Symptoms such as unexplained flashing lights or visual disturbances, transient numbness, unexplained bouts of abdominal pain or nausea, etc., all of which are considered to be fragments of a full-blown migraine attack. Migraine equivalents tend to occur most commonly in either children or older persons. Other disorders that might explain these symptoms must be ruled out by appropriate tests.

Migraineur - A designation sometimes used for people with migraine.

Monoamine Oxidase - A family of enzymes involved in the breakdown of certain neurotransmitters. MAO inhibitors act to block these enzymes.

MRI - An acronym for "magnetic resonance imaging", a computerized way of making pictures or images without the use of X-rays, but instead with the help of a powerful magnet.

MSG - Abbreviation for "monosodium glutamate", often found in seasonings or Chinese food. MSG may sometimes trigger migraine attacks in susceptible individuals.

Mineral: An inorganic substance. The major minerals in the body are calcium, phosphorus, potassium, sulfur, sodium, chloride, and magnesium.

Mucous membranes: Moist tissues forming the lining of body cavities that have an external opening, such as the respiratory, digestive, and urinary tracts.

Muscle Response Testing (MRT) or Neuromuscular testing (NST): A testing technique based on kinesiology to test allergies by comparing the strength of a muscle or a group of muscles in the presence and absence of the allergen.

NAR Foundation (NARF): A nonprofit research foundation dedicated to conduct research in allergy elimination of food, chemicals, environmental and other substances using NAET

NAET: (Nambudripad's Allergy Elimination Techniques): A technique to permanently eliminate allergies towards the treated allergens. Developed by Dr. Devi S. Nambudripad and practiced by more than 9,000 medical practitioners worldwide. This technique is natural, non-invasive, and drug-free. It has been effectively used in treating all types of allergies and problems arising from allergies. It is taught by Dr. Nambudripad in Buena Park, California. to currently licensed medical practitioners. If you are a licensed medical practitioner, interested in learning more about NAET, or NAET seminars, please visit the website: www.naet.com.

Naproxen - A nonsteroidal anti-inflammatory medication.

Narcotics - Strong prescription painkillers such as Demerol, Stadol, or Codeine, all of which are habit-forming if taken too often for too long at a time.

Naturopathy - The practice of the use of natural substances to provide a healthier balance of internal chemistry.

Neuralgia - The pain spasms of a major nerve. The pain can be jabbing, sudden and repetitive. There are several different types of neuralgia's, and each affects a different area. Trigeminal neuralgia, for example, affects the nerves of the face.

Neurologic - Relating to neurology or to the nervous system itself.

Say Good-bye to Headaches

Neurologist - A medical specialist with advanced training in diagnosis and treatment of diseases of the brain, spinal cord, nerves and muscles, including such common disorders as headache, dizziness, stroke and back pain.

Neurology - The branch of medical science that specializes in the nervous system.

Neurotransmitters - Naturally occurring chemicals in the brain which transmit messages from one nerve cell to another.

Neurovascular - Pertaining to the relationship between nerves and the blood vessels they supply.

Nitrites - Chemical preservatives used in meats, various processed foods and, because they are known to dilate blood vessels, they can cause headaches in some people.

Nondrug Therapy - A treatment that does not involve the use of drugs or medications. In the case of headache, such nondrug therapies might include: biofeedback, acupuncture, dietary counseling, stress management training, physical therapy, etc.

Nervous system: A network made up of nerve cells, the brain, and the spinal cord, which regulates and coordinates body activities.

NST: Neuromuscular testing (NST): A testing technique based on kinesiology to test allergies by comparing the strength of a muscle or a group of muscles in the presence and absence of the allergen.

NTT: A series of standard diagnostic tests used by NAET practitioners to detect allergies is called "Nambudripad's Testing Techniques" or NTT.

Neurotransmitter: A molecule that transmits electrical and/or chemical messages from nerve cell (neuron) to nerve cell or from nerve cell to muscle, secretory, or organ cells.

Nutrients: Vitamins, minerals, amino acids, fatty acids, and sugar (glucose), which are the raw materials needed by the body to provide energy, effect repairs, and maintain functions.

Ocular Migraine - A type of migraine with aura or "classical" migraine in which visual symptoms are prominent, sometimes with little or no headache component.

Glossary

Ophthalmoplegic Migraine - A very rare type of migraine in which there is weakness of one or more of the muscles that moves the eye. This is said to occur mainly in young people, and other, more common causes for painful paralysis of the eye muscles, must be excluded by appropriate diagnostic testing.

Organic foods: Foods grown in soil free of chemical fertilizers, and without pesticides, fungicides and herbicides.

Outgasing: The releasing of volatile chemicals that evaporate slowly and constantly from seemingly stable materials such as plastics, synthetic fibers, or building materials.

Overload: The overpowering of the immune system due to numerous concurrent exposures or to continuous exposure caused by many stresses, including allergens.

Oxygen Therapy - Breathing of oxygen from a tank which is sometimes very helpful for cluster headaches.

Pain Rating System - Since pain is an internal and private experience, various scales have been devised for rating pain. One of the most common, rates pain on a zero to ten scale, with ten being the most severe pain a person has ever experienced. Yet another assigns the number one to mild pain, two to moderate pain, three to severe pain, and four to pain that causes incapacity.

Parasite: An organism that depends on another organism (host) for food and shelter, contributing nothing to the survival of the host.

Pathogenic: Capable of causing disease.

Pathology: The scientific study of disease; its cause, processes, structural or functional changes, developments and consequences.

Pathway: The metabolic route used by body systems to facilitate biochemical functions.

Personality - In the past, it was thought that there was a typical "migraine personality". Now, this is no longer felt to be the case, as the primary factor determining whether or not a person will have migraine or not is heredity, not personality. Nevertheless, hurrying, worrying, and stress can all aggravate migraine.

Petrochemical: A chemical derived from petroleum or natural gas.

Say Good-bye to Headaches

pH: A scale from 1 to 14 used to measure acidity and alkalinity of solutions. A pH of 1-6 is acidic; a pH of 7 is neutral; a pH of 8-14 is alkaline or basic.

Postnasal drip: The leakage of nasal fluids and mucus down into the back of the throat.

Precursor: Anything that precedes another thing or event, such as physiologically inactive substance that is converted into an active substance that is converted into an active enzyme, vitamin, or hormone.

Prostaglandin: A group of unsaturated, modified fatty acids with regulatory functions.

Phonophobia - Abnormal sensitivity to sound.

Phosphenes - Tiny, brilliant sparks often seen during the first stage of migraine.

Photophobia - Abnormal sensitivity to light.

Postdrome - The period following a bad migraine headache during which a person feels "hung over", tired, and "beaten up" is referred to as the headache postdrome.

Posttraumatic Headache - Headache which follows an injury or trauma. There does not have to be loss of consciousness for an injury to cause significant headache in some cases.

Premenstrual Syndrome - (PMS) Combination of symptoms experienced by some women prior to menstruation.

Prodrome - The period of time preceding a migraine headache during which a person may feel irritable, out of sorts, moody, unusually sensitive to light or noise, and may notice some fluid retention. This may go on for one or two days or just a few hours before the actual headache begins.

Prophylactic Medication - Preventative medication taken on a regular schedule to prevent the onset of an ailment such as migraine.

Prophylaxis - Measures taken to prevent the development of headache. These measures may include daily use of medication or nondrug therapies.

Propranolol - Beta blocker medication widely prescribed for hypertension and other chronic conditions, and effective in preventing migraine.

Radiation: The process of emission, transmission, and absorption of any type of waves or particles of energy, such as light, radio, ultraviolet or X-rays.

Receptor: Special protein structures on cells where hormones, neurotransmitters, and enzymes attach to the cell surface.

Respiratory system: The system that begins with the nostrils and extends through the nose to the back of the throat and into the larynx and lungs.

Rebound Headache - A chronic form of headache brought about by taking painkillers to excess (usually at least two days out of three). This is thought to be due to suppression of the body's own painfighting mechanisms.

Referred Pain - Pain perceived as occurring in a part of the body other than its true source.

Scintillation - The perception of twinkling light of varying intensity that can occur during the migraine aura.

Scotoma - An area of decreased or lost vision. Scotoma can be a characteristic symptom of migraine auras.

Sensitivity: An adaptive state in which a person develops a group of adverse symptoms to the environment, either internal or external. Generally refers to non-IgE reactions.

Serotonin: A constituent of blood platelets and other organs that is released during allergic reactions. It also functions as a neurotransmitter in the body. Serotonin thought to be important in the mechanism of migraine headaches.

Sinus Headache - A headache caused by a clogged sinus cavity.

Sinusitis - Infection or inflammation of the sinuses. When the sinuses are infected, there is usually a low-grade fever, tenderness to touch over the sinuses, and a thick, colored nasal or post-nasal drainage.

Status Migrainosus - A severe unrelenting migraine headache associated with nausea and vomiting which lasts for several days and may not be manageable under outpatient care.

Stress - An emotionally disruptive or upsetting condition occurring in

Say Good-bye to Headaches

response to adverse external influences and capable of affecting physical health which can be characterized by increased heart rate, a rise in blood pressure, muscular tension, irritability and depression. Stress does not cause migraine but can be a migraine "trigger".

Sublingual: Under the tongue–method of testing or treatment in which a measured amount of an antigen or extract is administered under the tongue, behind the teeth. Absorption of the substance is rapid in this way.

Supplement: Nutrient material taken in addition to food in order to satisfy extra demands, effect repair, and prevent degeneration of body systems.

Susceptibility: An alternative term used to describe sensitivity.

Symptoms: A recognizable change in a person's physical or mental state, that is different from normal function, sensation, or appearance and may indicate a disorder or disease.

Syndrome: A group of symptoms or signs that, occurring together, produce a pattern typical of a particular disorder.

Synthetic: Made in a laboratory; not normally produced in nature, or may be a copy of a substance made in nature.

Systemic: Affecting the entire body.

Synapse - The junction between nerve cells where a nerve impulse is transferred from one neuron to another.

Syncope - A brief loss of consciousness (a blackout).

Temporal Arteritis - A headache caused by inflamed arteries in the head and neck. It requires immediate medical attention.

Tension Headache - As defined by the International Headache Society, a tension type headache is just the opposite of migraine. That is, the pain is on both sides of the head, is pressing and steady, rather than pulsating, is usually mild and does not cause incapacity and, is not worsened by ordinary daily activities. There is no associated nausea or sensitivity to light and noise.

TMJ - Acronym for "temporomandibular joint", or the joints where the jaw attaches to the skull just in front of the ears. It is sometimes linked to headache pain.

Toxicity: A poisonous, irritating, or injurious effect resulting when a person ingests or produces a substance in excess of his or her tolerance threshold.

Trigger - Anything that can set off a migraine headache in a genetically predisposed individual is referred to as a "trigger". Common triggers include (but are not limited to) stress, changes in female hormone levels, skipping meals, certain odors such as perfume, sleeping late on weekends, sleep loss, alcohol, and some foods including cheese, chocolate and MSG.

Trigeminal Nerve - The fifth cranial nerve, a major nerve of the face and head. It is related to nerve impulses that direct the muscles for jaw movement.

Tumor Headache - A headache caused by a tumor, or growth, that presses on the brain. Symptoms can include seizures, loss of consciousness, projectile vomiting and speech disturbances. While migraine sufferers can experience severe pain (making them feel as though they may have a tumor), of those persons suffering from migraine, less than 0.004% actually suffer from a brain tumor.

Tyramine - A substance found in meats, cheese and red wine, which can trigger migraine in a susceptible individual.

Unilateral - Affecting or relating to only one side.

Vascular - Relating to the channels that carry body fluids, usually used in connection with the blood vessels.

Vascular Pain - Pain caused by the dilation or constriction of blood vessels. Dilating (enlarging) the blood vessels in the head causes pain when the vessels exert pressure on surrounding nerves. Constructing (narrowing) the blood vessels reduces the supply of blood to the brain. The tissue around the blood vessels may become inflamed, and chemical irritants build up in the area.

Vasoactive - Affecting the dilation or constriction of blood vessels.

Verapamil - A type of calcium channel blocker medication which can be effective in preventing migraine.

Vertigo - The sensation of spinning or whirling. Resources

RESOURCES

www.naet.com - The NAET website for
information regarding NAET

Nambudripad Allergy Research Foundation (NARF)
6714 Beach Blvd.
Buena Park, CA 90621
(714) 523-0800
A Nonprofit foundation dedicated to NAET research

NAET Seminars
6714 Beach Blvd.
Buena Park, CA 90621
(714) 523-8900
NAET Seminar information

Delta Publishing Company (for Books on NAET)
6714 Beach Blvd.
Buena Park, CA 90621
(714) 523-0800
E-mail: naet@earthlink.net

Jacob Teitelbaum MD
CFS/Fibromyalgia Therapies
Author of the best selling book:
"From Fatigued to Fantastic!" and
"Three Steps to Happiness! Healing Through Joy"
(410) 573-5389
www.EndFatigue.com

Environmentally Safe Products
Quantum Wellness Center
Drs. Dave & Steven Popkin
1261 South Pine Island Rd.
Plantation, FL 33324
(954) 370-1900/ Fax: (954) 476-6281
E-mail: buddha327@aol.com

Cotton Gloves and other Environmentally
 Safe Health Products
 Janice Corporation
198 US Highway 46
Budd Lake, NJ 07828-3001
(800) 526-4237

Herbal Supplements
Kenshin Trading Corporation
1815 West 213th Street, Ste. 180
Torrance, CA 90501
(310) 212-3199

Phenolics
Frances Taylor/Dr. Jacqueline Krohn
Los Alamos Medical Center, Ste.136
3917 West Road
Los Alamos, NM 87544
(505) 662-9620

Enzyme Formulations, Inc
6421 Enterprise Lane
Madison, WI 53719
(800) 614-4400

Say Good-bye to Headaches

Bio Meridian
12411 S. 265 W. Ste. F
Draper, UT 84020
(801) 501-7517
Computerized Allergy Testing Services

Star Tech Health Services, LLC
1219 South 1840 West
Orem, Utah 84058
(888) 229-1114
Computerized Allergy Testing Services

Thorne Research Inc.
P.O. Box 25
Denver, ID 83825
(208) 263-1337
Herbs and Vitamins

K & T Books
LAMC, Ste. 136,
3917 West Road
Los Alamos, NM 87544
(505) 662 9620

Neuropathways EEG Imaging
427 North Canon Dr. # 209
Beverly Hills, CA 90210
(310) 276 9181

BIBLIOGRAPHY

Abehsera, Michel, Ed., *Healing Ourselves,* 1973

Ali, Majid M.D., *The Canary and Chronic Fatigue,* Life Span Press, 1995

American Medical Association Committee on Rating of Mental and Physical Impairments, *Guides to the Evaluation of Permanent Impairment,* N.P., 1971

American Psychiatric Association, *Diagnostic and Statistical Manual of Mental Disorders,* 4th. ed., 2000

Andress, E. and J. Harrison. 1999. *Flavored Vinegars. In 'So Easy to Preserve'.* 4th Ed. Cooperative Extension Service, The University of Georgia. 140-143.

Austin, Mary, *Acupuncture Therapy,* 1972

Baxter, R. and W. Holzapfel. 1982. A microbial investigation of selected spices, herbs, and additives in South Africa. J. Food Sc. 47:570-574.

Beckmann, G., D. Koszegi, B. Sonnenschein and R. Leimbeck. 1996. On the microbial status of herbs and spices. Fleischwirtschaft. 76(3): 240-243.

Beeson, Paul B., M.D. and McDermott, Walsh, M.D., Eds., *Textbook of Medicine,* 12th edition, 1967

Bender, David, and Bruno Leone, *The Environment, Opposing Viewpoints,* Greenhaven Press, 1996

Blum, Jeanne Elizabeth, *Woman Heal Thyself,* Charles E. Tuttle Co., 1995

Brodal, A., M.D., *Neurological Anatomy in Relation to Clinical Medicine,* 2nd ed.

Brownstein, David, *"Overcoming Arthritis"* Medical Alternatives press, 2001

Brownstein, David, *"Hormones and Chronic Disease"* Medical Alternatives press, 1999

Brownstein, David, *"The Miracle of Natural Hormones*, 1998. 152pp. Medical Alternatives Press. Author: *The Miracle of Natural Hormones* 2nd Edition. 1999. Medical Alternatives Press

Cecil Textbook Of Medicine, 21st ed., 2000

Cerrat, Paul L., *"Does Diet Affect the Immune System?"* RN, Vol. 53, pp. 67-70 (June 1990)

Chaitow, Leon, *The Acupuncture Treatment of Pain,* Thomsons Publishers, 1984

Chernoff, Marilyn, Daily dose of toxin,1924 Juan Tabo NE, Ste A, Albuquerque, NM 87112, 2006

Collins, Douglas, R. M.D., *Illustrated Diagnosis of Systematic Diseases,* 1972

Cousins, Norman, *Head First, The Biology of Hope and the Healing Power of the Human Spirit,* Penguin Books, 1990

Daniels, Lucille, M.A, and Catherine Wothingham, Ph.D., *Muscle Testing Techniques of Manual Examination,* 3rd ed., 1972

Davis, Rowland H., and Weller, Stephen G., *The Gist of Genetics,* Jones and Bartlett Publishers, 1996

East Asian Medical Studies Society, *Fundamentals of Chinese Medicine,* Paraadigm Publications, 1985

Elliot, Frank, A., F.R.C.P., *Clinical Laboratory*, 1959

Fazir, Claude A., M.D., *Parents Guide to Allergy in Children,* Doubleday & Co., 1973

FDA - CFSAN. 1998. *Guide to minimize microbial food safety hazards for fresh fruits and vegetables. At* http://www.cfsan.fda.gov/~dms/prodguid.html.

Fratkin, Jake, *Chinese Herbal Pattent Formulas,* Institute of Traditional Medicine, 1986

Fujihara, Ken and Hays, Nancy, *Common Health Complaints,* Oriental Healing Arts Institute, 1982

Fulton, Shaton, *The Allergy Self Help Book,* Rodale Books, 1983

Gabriel, Ingrid, *Herb Identifier and Handbook,* Sterling Publishing Co., 1980

Gach, Michael Reed, *Acuppressure's Potent Points,* Bantam Books, 1990

Goldberg, Burton and Eds. of Alternative Medicine Digest, *Chronic Fatigue and Fibromyalgia & Environmental Illness*, Future Medicine Publishing, 1998

Goldberg, Burton and Eds. of Alternative Medicine Digest, *Definitive Guide to Headaches,* Future Medicine Publishing, 1997

Golos, Natalie, and Frances, *Coping With Your Allergies,* Simon and Schuster

Goodheart, George, J., *Applied Kinesiology,* N.P., 1964

---. *Applied Kinesiology*, 1970 Research Manual, 8th ed. N.P., 1971

---. *Applied Kinesiology*, 1973 Research Manual, 9th ed. N.P., 1973

---. *Applied Kinesiology*, 1974 Research Manual, N.P., 1974

---.*Applied Kinesiology*, Workshop Manual, N.P., 1972

Gray, Henry, F.R.S., *Anatomy of the Human Body,* 27th, 34th, and 38th eds., 1961

Graziano, Joseph, *Footsteps to Better Health*, N.P., 1973

Guyton, Arthur C., *Textbook of Medical Physiology,* 2nd ed., 1961

Haldeman, Scott, *Modern Developments in the Principles and Practice of Chiropractic,* Appleton-Century-Crofts, 1980

Hansel, Tim, *When I Relax I Feel Guilty,* Chariot Victor Publishing, 1979

Harris H. M.D., and Debra Fulghum Bruce, *The Fibromyalglia Handbook*, Holt and Co., 1996

Hepler, Opal, E., Ph.D., M.D., *Manual of Clinical Laboratory Methods,* 4th ed., 1962

Heuns, Him-Che., *Handbook of Chinese Herbs and Formulae,* Vol V., 1985

Hsu, Hong-Yen, Ph.D., *Chinese Herb Medicine and Therapy,* Oriental Healing Arts Institute, 1982

---. *Commonly Used Chinese Herb Formulas with Illustrations,* Oriental Healing Arts Institute, 1982

---. *Natural Healing With Chinese Herbs,* Oriental Healing Arts Institute, 1982

Janeway, Charles A., and Travers, Paul, and Walport, Mark, and Shlomchik, Mark, *Immunobiology*, Garland Publishing, 2001

Jusleth, R. and R. Deibel. 1974. Microbial profile of selected spices and herbs at import. J. Milk Food Technol. 37 (8): 414-419.

Kandel, Schwartz, Jessell, *Principles of Neural Science,* McGraw Hill, 4th ed., 2000

Kennington & Church, *Food Values of Portions Commonly Used,* J.B. Lippincott Company, 1998

Kirschmann J.D. with Dunne, L.J., *Nutrition Almanac,* 2nd ed., McGraw Hill Book Co., 1984

Krohn, Jacqueline, M.D., and Taylor, Frances A., M.A. and Larson, Erla Mae, R.N., *Allergy Relief and Prevention*, 2nd. ed, Hartley & Marks, 1996

Krohn, Jacqueline, M.D., and Taylor, Frances A., M.A., *Natural Detoxification,* 2nd. ed, Hartley & Marks, 2000

Lawson-Wood, Denis, F.A.C.A. and Lawson-Wood, Joyce, *The Five Elements of Acupuncture and Chinese Massage,* 2nd ed., 1973

Lyght, Charles E., M.D., and John M. Trapnell, M.D., Eds., *The Merck Manual,* 11th ed., Merck Research Laboratories, 1966

MacKarness, Richard, *The Hazards of Hidden Allergies,* Mc Ilwain

Merkel, Edward K., and John, David T., and Krotoski, Wojciech A., Eds., Medical Parasitology, 8th. ed., W.B.Saunders Company, 1999

Milne, Robert, M.D., and More, Blake, and Goldberg, Burton, An Alternative Medicine Definitive Guide to Headaches, 1997

Mindell, Earl, Vitamin Bible, Warner Books, 1985.

Moss, Louis, M.D., Acupuncture and You, 1964

Moyers, Bill, Healing and the Mind, Doubleday, 1976

Nambudripad, DS: *NAET® Protocols and Procedures-part 1,* The Journal of NAET Energetics and Complementary Medicine, 2005, Vol. (1) (1), pp.17-25.NAET Center, Buena Park, CA, 2005.

Nambudripad, DS: *NAET® Protocols and Procedures-part 2,* The Journal of NAET Energetics and Complementary Medicine, 2005, Vol. (1)(2), pp.107-112.NAET Center, Buena Park, CA.

Nambudripad, DS: *NAET® Protocols and Procedures-part 3,* The Journal of NAET Energetics and Complementary Medicine, Vol. (1)(3), pp.179-184. NAET Center, Buena Park, CA, 2005.

Nambudripad, DS: *NAET® Protocols and Procedures-part 4,* The Journal of NAET Energetics and Complementary Medicine, 2005, Vol. (1) (4), pp.265-270. NAET Center, Buena Park, CA.

Nambudripad, DS: *NAET® Protocols and Procedures-part 5,* The Journal of NAET Energetics and Complementary Medicine, Vol. (2)(1), pp.343-350. NAET Center, Buena Park, CA, 2005.

Nambudripad, Devi, *Living Pain Free,* Delta Publishing Company, 1997

Nambudripad, Devi, *Say Good-bye to ADD and ADHD,* Delta Publishing Company, 1999

Nambudripad, Devi, *Say Good-bye to Allergy-related Autism,* Delta Publishing Company, 1999

Nambudripad, Devi, *Say Good-bye to Children's Allergies,* Delta Publishing Company, 2000

Nambudripad, Devi, *Say Good-bye to Environmental Allergies,* Delta Publishing Company, 2002

Nambudripad, Devi, *Say Good-bye to Chemical Sensitivities,* Delta Publishing Company, 2002

Nambudripad, Devi, *Survivimg Biohazard Agents,* Delta Publishing Company, 2002

Nambudripad, Devi, *The NAET Guidebook,* Delta Publishing Company, 2001

Northrup, Christiane M.D., *Women's Bodies, Women's Wisdom,* Bantam Books, 1998

Palos, Stephan, *The Chinese Art of Healing,* 1972

Pearson, Durk, and Shaw, Sandy, *The Life Extension Companion,* Warner Books, 1984

Pert, Candace B., Ph.D., *Molecules of Emotion,* Scribner, 1997

Pitchford, Paul, *Healing with Whole Foods,* North Atlantic Books, 1993

Powers, E., R. Lawyer and Y. Masuoka. 1975. *Microbiology of Processed spices. J. Milk Food Technol.* 39 (11): 683-687.

Radetsky, Peter, *Allergic to the Twentieth Century,* Boston, Little, Brown and Co., 1997

Randolph, Theron, G., M.D., and Ralph W. Moss, Ph.D., *An Alternative Approach to Allergies,* Lippincott and Conwell, 1980

Rapp, Doris, *Allergy and Your Family,* Sterling Publishing Co., 1980

Rapp, Doris, *Is This Your Child?* Quill, William Morrow, 1991

Shanghai College of Traditional Chinese, *Acupuncture, a Comprehensive Text*

Shealy, C. Norman, M.D., Ph. D. and Caroline Myss, Ph. D., *The Creation of Health,* Stillpoint Publishing, 1993

Shima, Mike, *The Medical I Ching,* Blue Poppy Press, 1992

Shubert, Charlotte "Burned by FlameRretardants?" SCIENCE NEWS Vol. 160 (October 13, 2001), pgs. 238-239.

Sierra, Ralph, U., *Chiropractic Handbook of Applied Neurology,* Mexico, 1956

Somekh, Emile, M.D. *The Complete Guide To Children's Allergies,* Pinnacle Books, Inc. 1979

Smith, CW, Electromagnetic Man: *Health and Hazard in the Electrical Environment,* Martin's Press, 1989, 90, 97

Smith CW, Environmental Medicine: *Electromagnetic Aspects of Biological Cycles,* 1995:9(3):113-118

Smith CW., *Electrical Environmental Influences on the Autonomic Nervous System,* 11th. Intl. Symp. on *"Man and His Environment in Health and Disease",* Dallas, Texas, February 25-28,1993

Smith CW., *Electromagnetic Fields and the Endocrine System,* 10th. Intl. Symp. on *"Man and His Environment in Health and Disease",* Dallas Texas, February 27- March 1, 1992

Smith CW., *Basic Bioelectricity: Bioelectricity and Environmental Medicine,* 15th. Intl. Symp., on *"Man and His Environment in Health and Disease",* Dallas, Texas, February 20-23, 1997. (Audio Tapes from: Professional Audio Recording, 2300 Foothill Blvd. #409, La Verne, CA

Smith, John, H., D.C., *Applied Kinesiology and the Specific Muscle Balancing Technique.*

Say Good-bye to Headaches

J.E. Teitelbaum, B. Bird, R.M. Greenfield, et al., *"Effective Treatment of CFS and FMS: A Randomized, Double-Blind Placebo Controlled Study,"* Journal of Chronic Fatigue Syndrome 8 (2) (2001).

Teitlebaum, Jacob, M.D.,*Three Steps to Happiness!* 1st ed., 2001, Avery Penguin Putnam

Teitlebaum, Jacob, M.D.,*Healing through Joy"* 1st ed., 2002, Avery Penguin Putnam

Teitlebaum, Jacob, M.D.,*Pain Pain Go Away !*1st ed., 2003, 2nd. ed., 2001, Avery Penguin Putnam

Sui, Choa Kok, *Pranic Healing*, Samuel Wiser, 1990

Weiss, Jordan, M.D., *Psychoenergetics,* 2nd. ed., Oceanview Publishing, 1995

Zong, Linda, *"Chinese Internal Medicine,"* lectures at SAMRA University, Los Angeles, 1985

Case Histories from the Author's private practice,1984-present

INDEX

Say Good-bye to Headaches

Index

Say Good-bye to Headaches

Index

Say Good-bye to Headaches

About The Author

Devi S. Nambudripad, M.D., D.C., L.Ac., Ph.D. (Acu.)

Born in India, Dr. Devi S. Nambudripad has made California her home since 1976. In an effort to solve her personal health problems suffered since childhood, and to help others with similar problems, she conducted research in the United States over the past twenty years resulting in the development of a new and effective approach, known as Nambudripad's Allergy Elimination Techniques (NAET®), for diagnosis and treatment of allergies of all types.

She has pointed the way to perfect health by combining many methods and techniques from different disciplines of medicine, including: Allopathic, Kinesiology, Chiropractic, and Oriental medical procedures of Acupuncture and Acupressure. Dr. Nambudripad has received extensive training in each of these fields both in the United States and in the Orient.

To date, thousands of patients who could not find relief elsewhere have been successfully treated for both food and environmental allergies by NAET. Dr. Nambudripad has trained thousands of medical professionals in her special procedure on permanent allergy elimination. NAET training seminars are open to currently licensed medical practitioners. Any licensed doctors interested in finding out more about NAET training, please call or write to:

> NAET® Seminars
> 6714 Beach Blvd., Buena Park, CA 90621
> Tel: (714) 523-8900, email: naet@earthlink.net

An internationally known lecturer, Dr. Nambudripad has been a guest speaker at conferences, as well as, on radio and television. Her recently published books "Say Good-Bye To Illness," "Living Pain Free with Acupressure," "The NAET Guide Book," and the "Say Good-Bye To..." series.are available from:

> Delta Publishing Company
> 6714 Beach Blvd., Buena Park, CA 90621
> Tel: (888) 890-0670 / (714) 523-8900
> Fax: (714) 523-3068
> website: http://www.naet.com

SAY GOOD-BYE TO HEADACHES

Nambudripad's Testing Technique gave me the best tool to evaluate my patients' health disorders, and NAET taught me the greatest healing technique to eliminate headaches almost instantly and painlessly. NAET has truly revolutionized the practice of medicine! I applaud Dr. Devi for developing this unique technique and sharing with the world. I have no doubt this is going to be the Medicine of the Future.
Robert Prince, M.D. • Charlotte, NC

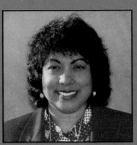

Devi S. Nambudripad,
M.D., D.C., L.Ac., Ph.D. (Acu.)

Dr. Devi's method has brought the understanding and approach to healing to a deeper level. It still puzzles me everyday how easily and thoroughly my patients are relieved of migraines and other types of headaches and can enjoy a healthy life again or, in some cases, experience it for the first time. There is no turning back now. Medicine can only progress from here.
Frederique Nault, N.D. • Bali, Indonesia

If you have ever had a persistent headache, you can understand what chronic pain feels like. Chronic pains became a major part of my life a few years ago in the form of headaches. I haven't had any more headaches after clearing the NAET basic fifteen. I am so thankful to God that I was guided to NAET.
Dr. Mary Sural • Orange, California

In our years of working with NAET, my wife and I have been repeatedly amazed at the medical conditions that improve with this therapy. It has been especially effective in those illnesses that most physicians are poorly trained in. Getting pain relief is one of these. You don't have to be in pain anymore!
Jacob Teitelbaum, M.D. • Annapolis, Maryland

For more information, please visit our website:
http://www.naet.com

Price: $18.00 US $24.00 CAN

ISBN-13: 978-0-9759277-6-2
ISBN-10: 0-9759277-6-0

NAMBUDRIPAD'S ALLERGY ELIMINATION TECHNIQUES
NAET®

51800

9 780975 927762